"*Essentials of Medical Intuition* brings groundbreaking research in medical intuition and proposes a new paradigm for the future of healthcare. Wendie Colter's dedication to helping us recognize the value of medical intuition and its inclusion into healthcare and further scientific research will define the use of this important skill for decades to come."

Paul J. Mills, PhD, Professor, Family Medicine and Public Health, Director of the Center of Excellence for Research and Training in Integrative Health, University of California, San Diego

"Wendie Colter is an extraordinary guide, helping us explore, understand and appreciate the wondrous gifts and potential of medical intuition, a new frontier in healthcare. *Essentials of Medical Intuition* shows us simply and practically how to cultivate our intuition for our own personal growth and to benefit those we serve. Filled with scientific research, case studies and guidance, it is an important book for any healthcare professional interested in developing their intuitive abilities."

Lucia Thornton, ThD, RN, MSN, AHN-BC, Past President, American Holistic Nurses Association, Immediate Past Chair, Academy of Integrative Health & Medicine, author of *Whole Person Carings*

"We need to integrate medicine so people are not a diagnosis or a body part but are a story which needs to be heard and responded to. We need to include mind, dreams, intuition, mysticism, and images with the body in medical education. Colter's *Essentials of Medical Intuition* brings this expanded vision of healthcare to the forefront."

Bernie Siegel, MD, author of *Love, Medicine & Miracles* and *The Art of Healing*

"A fascinating journey through the concepts, current uses, and future possibilities of medical intuition. With compelling case studies and evidence-supported science, Wendie presents a convincing case for including medical intuition in healthcare training and education."

Hyla Cass, MD, Integrative Psychiatrist, author of *8 Weeks to Vibrant Health*

"There is a domain of knowing we all possess that lies beyond language, logic, and thought. Colter's book describes this natural ability and how to allow it to flower in our daily life"

Larry Dossey, MD, author of *One Mind*

"Colter describes how medical intuition, along with professional judgment, can reveal the intrinsic links between our life experiences, our beliefs, and our health, as well as the transformative possibilities of incorporating this unique skill into an effective, integrative approach to healthcare."

Kenneth R. Pelletier, PhD, MD, Clinical Professor of Medicine, author of
Change Your Genes, Change Your Life

"What a beautiful book about medical intuition this truly is ... Wendie Colter reminds us all of the 'art' of medicine – an essential yet oft-neglected consideration. I hope that in the future, universities will be able to add this important component of medicine to their curricula."

Dominique Fradin-Read, MD, MPH

"In her clear, concise, and practical book, Wendie Colter envisions medical intuition assessment as fully integrated into whole-person wellness as a way to help address ongoing systemic crises in healthcare. She also provides specific self-directed intuitive instructions for your mind, body and spirit."

Lori Chortkoff Hops, PhD, DCEP, Licensed Psychologist, Educator,
President, Association for Comprehensive Energy Psychology

"Colter scientifically affirms that the intuitive nature of wellbeing is present in everyone, and that the role of the certified medical intuitive is to identify and facilitate the emergence of innate information to heal mind, body and spirit."

Gilah Yelin Hirsch, MFA, Professor of Art Emerita, California State
University Dominguez Hills (Los Angeles), multidisciplinary artist, author,
filmmaker, theorist

"One of Colter's most important messages is that healthcare professionals can and should be trained to develop 'intuitive assessment' skills. Such information merits consideration along with evidence from clinical trials and clinical experience of whole-person care."

Richard Hammerschlag, PhD, Nova Institute Scholar, Co-Director of Research
at the Consciousness and Healing Initiative (CHI), Dean Emeritus
of Research at the Oregon College of Oriental Medicine

ESSENTIALS OF
MEDICAL
INTUITION

A VISIONARY PATH TO WELLNESS

WENDIE COLTER

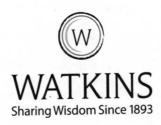

WATKINS
Sharing Wisdom Since 1893

This edition first published in the UK and USA in 2022 by
Watkins, an imprint of Watkins Media Limited
Unit 11, Shepperton House
89–93 Shepperton Road
London
N1 3DF

enquiries@watkinspublishing.com

Design and typography copyright © Watkins Media Limited 2022

Text copyright © Wendie Colter 2022

10 9 8 7 6 5 4 3 2 1

Typeset by Lapiz

Printed and bound in the UK by TJ Books Ltd.

A CIP record for this book is available from the British Library

ISBN: 978-1-78678-523-7 (Hardback)
ISBN: 978-1-78678-612-8 (eBook)

www.watkinspublishing.com

Publisher's note: The information presented in this book about medical intuition is educational in nature and is provided only as general information and is not medical or psychological advice nor is it intended as a substitute for licensed health care services. Although all of the case studies that are included in this book are true and based on factual situations, some information and identifying details have been changed to protect the identity of the individuals described. The author and publisher shall have neither responsibility nor liability to any person or entity with respect to any loss, damage, or injury caused or alleged to be caused directly or indirectly by the information contained in this book, including journal practices and exercises.

To Jimm, who makes my life happier every day,
and to my dearest Taj, who blooms like roses.

CONTENTS

Foreword   1

Introduction   5

Chapter 1   Developing Intuition   11

Chapter 2   What Is Medical Intuition?   25

Chapter 3   A Brief History of Medical Intuition   43

Chapter 4   Show Me the Evidence: Intuition
            in Healthcare   53

Chapter 5   Medical Intuition in Action: Establishing a
            New Paradigm   69

Chapter 6   The Mind–Body Connection   85

Chapter 7   The Energetics of Trauma   97

Chapter 8   Our Marvelous Meta-Senses   109

Chapter 9   Medical Intuition for Self-Care   127

Chapter 10 Seeing into the Future of Healthcare   141

Acknowledgments   153

About the Author   157

Endnotes   159

Index   189

FOREWORD

It was a beautiful day on Ruby Beach 25 years ago. I had just concluded a presentation at a medical meeting in Seattle, Washington, and traveled to the Olympic peninsula with my daughter, Hope, who was in her teens at the time. We were hiking along the beach, the ocean was calm, and I spotted a sea cave. Curiosity got the best of me as we hiked into the cave. I was engrossed in the intricacy of the structure when I suddenly had a violent foreboding feeling accompanied by a physical stress response. I screamed at my daughter to run out of the cave as fast as she could, and I followed suit. Within one minute of us clearing the cave, a rip tide struck with such force that the cave was quickly and completely filled with water, which sprayed at least 100ft into the air. Had I not experienced that sudden intuition, we would have perished. I was grateful, frightened and mystified by that event. The mystery and wonder of intuition has persisted with me since that day.

Having attended engineering school prior to medical school, I was a strict believer in the scientific basis of all natural phenomena ... until that day. The experience has served me well as I approach taking care of patients with a reverence of the mystery of human existence. There have been numerous instances when my intuition has been quite accurate when caring for others. I would venture to say that the vast majority of my colleagues would agree behind closed doors (perhaps we need to transform the cultural norm in order to appreciate and respect the mystery of life).

As fate would have it, my wife became friends with a woman who claimed to be a medical intuitive. As usual, I approached her claim with scientific skepticism until I encountered a patient with a fever of unknown origin. I was pleased to have found an underlying prostate infection, which can be difficult to diagnose. My satisfaction with having made the diagnosis was cut short as the patient's fever persisted, and I was at a loss. I called my wife's friend and gave her the name, birthdate and geographic location of the patient. She became quiet for a few minutes, and then said that she saw a "hot spot" in the pelvis and an additional "hot spot" in the area of the throat. I told her that the patient had no symptoms in the throat area, and she indicated that she was not a doctor but knew what she saw.

After a thorough evaluation of the throat from a medical viewpoint, I was then able to diagnose the patient with a rare condition – a silent inflammation of the thyroid gland. Ordinarily, one is unable to diagnose this condition in the absence of targeted tests as, despite inflammation, there is no tenderness upon palpation. Well, suffice it to say, my respect for her abilities skyrocketed, and I called upon her on several subsequent occasions when I was presented with a patient without a clear answer. I have been and remain respectful and continue to have reverence for the mystery of the process underlying the phenomenon of medical intuition.

Having come to firmly attest to the reality of this state, I had the good fortune to meet Wendie Colter through colleagues and subsequently in person at an integrative health conference in San Diego. It was my belief that individuals who were able to accurately see in a way that others could not, possess a rare gift. Wendie and I engaged in a discussion in which she indicated that she was able to teach the gift to healthcare professionals – a fact that shattered yet another belief. She not only has a training program but has published a definitive study in a respected, peer-reviewed journal, which is described in this book.

My ongoing discussions with Wendie have taught me that the gift of intuition is a gift to each and every human. Furthermore, my encounter with Wendie led me to develop a BioEnergy and Health Committee within the Integrative Health Policy Consortium, an organization devoted to the transformation of healthcare with focus on wellness and wellbeing (with the incorporation of scientifically valid, cost-effective approaches, such as medical intuition).

You have in your hands a valuable gift. This landmark book should be approached with an open mind and a willingness to expand your own understanding and knowledge of the mystery we call life, and that the indigenous peoples of the world have been trying to teach us for millennia. I have come to believe that to not believe in intuition is counterintuitive.

Thank you for this beautiful gift for us all, Wendie.

Leonard A. Wisneski, MD, FACP
Faculty: Georgetown University, George Washington University, University of Colorado
Chair Emeritus, Integrative Health Policy Consortium
Author: *The Scientific Basis of Integrative Health*

INTRODUCTION

Don't try to comprehend with your mind. Your minds are very limited. Use your intuition.

Madeleine L'Engle, *A Wind in the Door*

All great leaps forward in science and medicine begin with the willingness to imagine an unimaginable possibility. Bold new ideas in integrative healthcare are emerging in the synthesis of Western medicine and evidence-supported energy-based methods. Patients, clients and practitioners are looking for a multileveled, practical approach that can help heal not only the body but also the mind and spirit.

The illuminating skill of medical intuition is designed to provide fast, accurate intuitive health assessments that can be used as both a standalone practice and as a powerful support to healthcare of every kind. Medical intuition is intended to uncover the hidden sources of energetic resistance that may be blocking optimal health, and to create an essential and practical roadmap for full-spectrum wellbeing.

My intention in writing this book is to help people understand medical intuition – what it is, what it isn't – and how it can offer a comprehensive perspective for wellness in ways that conventional medicine cannot reach. Throughout this book, you will find a series of intuitive exercises intended to help you grow and develop your own inherent intuition.

I include fascinating case studies describing how medical intuitives help pinpoint the underlying drivers of illness, imbalance and disease. I explain how our bodies can hold energetic information hidden within our own life stories, our beliefs and our emotions that may have a significant impact on our health.

You will learn about the history and evolution of medical intuition, examine peer-reviewed research, discover current uses and get a glimpse into the future of this exciting and evolving field. You will read interviews with healthcare providers who work closely with medical intuitives and those who use medical intuition in their own practices. These health professionals have seen the benefits in their patients' and clients' outcomes, and they have no interest in going back to medicine-as-usual.

Let's begin with a few important caveats. First of all, this book is not a "how-to" manual on the use of medical intuition with your patients, clients or loved ones. I believe the best way to master the skill of medical intuition is in a focused educational environment with the guidance of an experienced and ethical instructor. Secondly, medical intuition is not defined as an energy healing method, such as Reiki or Healing Touch. Chapter 2 presents a formal definition of medical intuition, and clarifies how it is a distinct intuitive observational assessment process based on energetic "scanning" or "reading." And, finally, although this book is geared toward wellness professionals, it is also for everyone who is curious about medical intuition and would like to learn more.

In Chapter 3, you will meet some of the pioneers and thought leaders who created the foundations for modern medical intuition. Chapter 4 delves into the cutting-edge research in healthcare dedicated to exploring the boundaries of human intuition and how science is validating our innate intuitive abilities.

In Chapter 5, discover how talented medical intuitives and doctors work together in the clinical setting. These ground-breaking collaborations – some of which have never before been made public – demonstrate a successful new paradigm and vision for the future.

What roles do our own thoughts and feelings play in our health? The tenets of mind–body medicine are explored in

Chapter 6. I discuss the power of visualization and show how you can create a deeper intuitive connection with your own body.

Chapter 7 focuses on the energetics of trauma. I explain how medical intuition can reveal the messages hidden within our unique life history, how traumatic life events may affect our health, and the importance of "permission for wellness" in healing.

Our wonderful, natural intuitive "meta-senses" (also known as the *clairs*) are explored in depth in Chapter 8, along with some of the intriguing research behind them. I describe how we use our intuition every day, often without even realizing it. Best of all, you will have the opportunity to take your intuition for a spin with a set of focused exercises.

Chapter 9 offers useful tools for medical intuitive self-care, including a deep healing dialogue with your own body's wisdom. These specialized exercises are designed to build energetic resiliency and can be used daily.

For this book, I was honored to sit down with some of the legends and leading lights in intuitive health, and I am delighted to share their wisdom and vision. Chapter 10 presents a future of healthcare that embraces medical intuition in the hospital, the clinic and the classroom.

Some of you may enter this subject with enthusiasm and a desire to jump right in. For others, the term "medical intuition" might sound too "woo-woo." It's true that there are aspects of medical intuition that cannot always be easily explained. As you read this book, consider how your own intuition might enhance your wellness practice – for your patients, clients and for yourself. I believe that you will begin to understand the purpose and value of medical intuition.

As I have seen in my own practice of more than 20 years, incorporating intuition can make you a better practitioner. I have been fortunate to teach medical intuition to physicians, nurses, allied healthcare professionals, holistic healing arts practitioners and others. I have presented or taught at prominent education centers at the forefront of whole-person health, including the Academy of Integrative Health & Medicine (AIHM) Fellowship; the Andrew Weil Center for Integrative Medicine's Integrative Medicine Elective Rotation (IMER) program, University of Arizona, Tucson; Guarneri Integrative Health, Inc. at Pacific Pearl La Jolla, La Jolla, California; the American Holistic Nurses Association (AHNA); and the Association for Comprehensive Energy Psychology (ACEP), among others. I'm honored to serve on the Integrative Health Policy Consortium (IHPC) BioEnergy and Health Committee.

Before we dig in, I will start with my own story, and you'll read more about my personal journey within these pages. My path to medical intuition took many twists and turns, but intuition has always been there to help guide my way.

At a young age, I recall having fascinating metaphysical experiences. I remember powerful lucid dream adventures with detailed information about the nature of life on earth, karma, spiritual direction and more. As a teenager, a summer job at the Bodhi Tree, Los Angeles' iconic "new age" bookstore, gave me access to the many classics of spiritual thought. As I grew up, my intuition grew with me and I learned to trust it. Through a dear friend, I was introduced to affirmations and energy healing concepts at Louise Hay's renowned living-room gatherings in Santa Monica, California. I was blessed with many wise teachers who nurtured and encouraged my spiritual development. Intuition was always a source of wonder, education and fun.

For most of my life, I've been a professional musician. Starting out as a performer, I became a composer, publisher and executive producer in the high-powered corporate world of the music industry. Early on, while studying in music school and playing in rock bands, I visited a psychic who told me I was destined to be a "healer." When I told her that idea was miles away from my career goals, she said, "Music can be very healing, too. But at some point, you'll make a transition into healing full-time." I avoided that prediction for years.

In my music career, I sometimes felt like I was living a double life. After work, I immersed myself in studies of energy healing practices, spirituality, intuition and meditation. I graduated from the intuitive studies, energy medicine, ministerial, and teacher-training programs at a noted school of metaphysics in Los Angeles. I became an instructor of energy medicine and intuitive development, an ordained minister and a Master Certified Wellness Coach.

Medical intuition was something that developed naturally for me, over time. As I began my professional energy healing practice, I found I was able to intuitively *see* directly into the client's body, along with images of where, when and how a health issue had manifested. Inspired by positive feedback from my clients, I began to recognize the effectiveness of medical intuition. It became clear that healthcare, from the typical symptom-based Western medicine perspective, was simply not working as well as it could.

I saw a gap that medical intuition was uniquely designed to fill, and a place for my talents in teaching doctors, nurses and other wellness professionals to use this powerful knowledge. I created my accredited program, The Practical Path® Medical Intuitive Training™ Practitioner Certification Program, as a systematic method to access, develop and optimize intuition in order to address the deepest need for innovative intuitive skills. (See www.thepracticalpath.com, for more information.)

As a medical intuitive practitioner, I have seen that if the underlying emotional, mental and spiritual aspects of physical issues are not addressed, healing may be elusive at best – and, at worst, a cause of despair and failing health. As for practitioners themselves, it is evident that they need healing, too. Physicians and nurses are now speaking openly about their levels of burnout, frustration and disillusionment with the current medical systems, and are looking for more meaningful ways to practice.

My hope is that this book will assist in validating your own intuition. I also hope it will pique your curiosity to develop it further and provide more opportunities to help support vibrant wellbeing for your patients, your clients and for yourself.

To get started, here is an age-old question worth contemplating: Is healthcare an art, a science, or both? Albert Einstein said, "The most beautiful thing we can experience is the mysterious. It is the source of all true art and all science."[1] Medical intuition merges the art and science of healing, illuminating the beautiful and profound mysteries contained within.

CHAPTER 1

DEVELOPING INTUITION

The highest endeavor of the mind, and the highest virtue, is to understand things by intuition.

Baruch Spinoza

The skill of intuitive insight has been part of the human experience for millennia. Throughout history, oracles, sages and seers have used intuitive skills to help people interpret the deeper meanings hidden within the events of their lives. In every era and culture across the globe, those gifted with "second sight" were the trusted cornerstones of their communities, embodying the roles of healers, leaders and counselors.

Socrates wrote about an "inner voice" that gave him valuable instructions, which he claimed he could hear as clearly as any conversation.[1] Painters, poets, authors and musicians refer to their muse, a mercurial energy that overtakes them when deeply engaged in the creative process. Inventors, scientists and physicists, including Faraday, Kelvin, Gauss and Tesla, were familiar with Archimedes' eureka effect – a powerful "Aha!" moment of lucidity that brings sudden clarity and inspiration. Albert Einstein wrote, "It is not intellect, but intuition which advances humanity," and famously relied on frequent power naps to intuitively spark his scientific theories.[2] Many great thinkers and cultural leaders have also openly acknowledged the importance of intuition in their work and their lives, including physician Jonas Salk, inventor of the polio vaccine; psychologist

Carl G. Jung; media executive Oprah Winfrey; and entrepreneur Richard Branson.

Intuition permeates our lives. We may recognize it as gut feelings, hunches or uncanny, even illogical, occurrences of *knowing*, *feeling* or *sensing*. Although this may be new to you, intuition is being used every day by medical doctors, nurses and mental health therapists in hospitals, clinics and in private practice.[3] Holistic health providers, such as naturopathic doctors, acupuncturists, chiropractors, nutritionists and energy-based practitioners, may also use their intuition. These wellness professionals have that "special something" their patients and clients all seem to appreciate.

The word "intuition" comes from the Latin *intuitus*, meaning "to gaze at or contemplate." It is defined as "a direct perception of truth, fact … independent of any reasoning process."[4] Perhaps the reasoning process appears to be missing because our intuitive perceptions can't be pigeonholed into our five universally accepted senses of sight, smell, hearing, touch and taste. Intuition truly is our "sixth sense."

Misconceptions, Myths and Taboos

There is a great deal of misunderstanding about natural intuitive abilities in our modern world. When I discuss the misconceptions surrounding intuition with medical professionals, I ask them for the first image they think of when they hear the word "psychic." Take a moment to imagine in your mind's eye what you think of when you read that word.

For most people, the flashing neon sign of a storefront palm reader or the iconic image of a mystical woman with a crystal ball springs to mind. People are understandably wary of this kind of connotation, especially in the critical area of healthcare. Societal and cultural taboos have marginalized the field of intuitive development for centuries due to superstition, fears of charlatanism, religious stigma and passed-down cultural beliefs. Over the years, as the advancement of medical science has allowed us to enjoy longer and healthier lives, it has also ingrained the idea that its methods are the most rational and effective. As a result, anything claiming to support health that isn't part of mainstream medicine is likely to be considered ineffectual or fraudulent.

Yet when I ask wellness providers if they've ever acted on their intuition, even as a hunch or gut feeling about a patient or client's issues, which proved to be accurate, there are nods of recognition all around. Frequently, when I speak at health conferences, physicians, nurses and other healthcare professionals approach me to share their own extraordinary intuitive encounters in confidential, but excited, voices. Some tell me they have worked with a medical intuitive at least once in their practice, often to consult on a difficult case. Many want to learn more about how to grow and develop their own intuition. They are highly supportive of the need for more peer-reviewed science, transparency and acceptance of the skill.

It is important to remember that even a relatively short time ago, the topic of intuition would never have been deemed remotely appropriate for a healthcare conference. That we can now talk about intuition in a brightly lit conference hall and not huddled in a basement somewhere – the way doctors had to hide their discoveries in centuries past – I consider a major leap forward! But within the confines of typical conventional medicine environments, the atmosphere to discuss intuitive observations is still so stifled that most healthcare professionals are afraid to mention any of their experiences to colleagues.

It's not hard to understand their concerns. From my perspective, though, it is just as important to be open-minded as it is to be skeptical. After all, science is constantly evolving. What was once off-limits is now a key part of thoughtful, integrative care. For example, when combined with the advances of Western medicine, clinicians are seeing significant benefits for patients using holistic disciplines such as acupuncture, massage therapy, herbal medicine, whole-food nutrition and evidence-supported energy healing methods.[5] Even the United

States Veterans Administration has adopted a cutting-edge initiative called Whole Health, which incorporates meditation, nutrition, yoga and more.[6]

These innovative concepts are transforming healthcare by emphasizing a "whole-person" approach for physical, emotional, mental and spiritual health. In this new frontier, medical intuition has a fundamental role to play.

Aren't You Just Born With It?

"What's the symbol?" my sister asked, holding up a Zener card but hiding the image from my view. I scrunched up my face in an eight-year-old's approximation of deep concentration, trying to "receive" the image she was sending to me with her mind. "A circle?" I asked. "Right!" she exclaimed, and turned the card around to reveal a circle symbol. Then it was my turn to pick a card for her and the game continued. Even though I didn't always get the correct answer, it was thrilling when I did – and I loved the challenge either way.

Just as some children show an early aptitude for scholastic abilities such as math or sports, many display a natural talent for intuition. Parents and teachers usually encourage kids who excel in their favorite subjects. However, a child who excels in intuition may be shushed, thwarted or ignored because of a lack of understanding. This might even have been the case for you. That doesn't mean your intuition can't be re-ignited or even developed later in life. It just indicates that our society currently knows very little about the value of intuition.

In many ways, I was lucky. Intuition was not openly discussed in our home but it wasn't discouraged either. My mother, an artist, fostered an open and tolerant atmosphere for all creative pursuits. I found out much later that one of my mother's dear friends, the photographer Hella Hammid, who took beautiful pictures of our family, was also a renowned psychic. Hella worked with extrasensory perception (ESP) researcher Russell Targ on his experiments in remote viewing for the US government. She also accompanied researcher Stephan A. Schwartz on his archaeology endeavor, the Alexandria Project, where she helped to intuitively locate the ruins of the palace of Cleopatra and other phenomenal discoveries.

Zener cards were invented by perceptual psychologist Karl Zener and parapsychologist Joseph B. Rhine for their legendary ESP experiments at Duke University, North Carolina. I believe Hella gave me the Zener card set to provide quiet encouragement in developing my intuition. However, for many of the people I teach, intuition was not discussed or even understood in their upbringing.

People most often experience intuition as an intuitive "hit" when they least expect it. Without warning, like a bolt of lightning, we *sense*, *feel* or "get" information that we had no way of previously knowing. I call this having a "flash of insight" – a random moment of intuitive clarity. Flashes of insight are wonderful and can be quite profound. But they can also be unpredictable, unrepeatable and incomplete. You will learn that medical intuition is a systematic, deliberate method of asking for and receiving information, directly from both the physical body systems and the subtle energy systems of the body, also referred to as the "biofield" (*see* more in the "Biofield" section of this chapter).

Don't worry if you do not have any early intuitive memories or have never had a flash of intuitive insight. The ability is still there within you. Medical intuition may sound like an incredible superpower, but I believe intuition is a hardwired, natural human trait that anyone can develop and optimize into a practical and useful skill. Simply put, learning how to build your intuition is much like learning how to speak a new language, play an instrument or strengthen a muscle. It takes correct instruction, plenty of practice, and time. It isn't only for a select few or uniquely gifted individuals. We are *all* born with it.

The Spiritual Psyche and Health

Intuition may perhaps be best described as a way to access the interconnected nature of human consciousness. The term "nonduality," also known as "nonlocal" awareness, comes from the Sanskrit word *advaita*, meaning "non-separation."

Referred to as the quantum mind, entanglement, and even "cosmic soup," scientific evidence of nonlocality suggests that human consciousness is not confined to our minds or bodies, or even to specific moments in time.[7]

In the *Handbook of Complementary and Alternative Therapies in Mental Health*, psychiatrist Eric Leskowitz calls this nonlocal wisdom "transpersonal" intuition, a type of consciousness that operates "beyond the reach of the everyday personality, beyond the reach of the five physical senses, and beyond the limitations of space and time."[8] The metaphysical belief in a higher self, higher source, or soul, is another way to frame this intuitive connection.

Sadly, our spiritual nature has long been ignored by biomedicine as a factor in health and healing. In 380 BCE, Plato wrote, "This is the great error of our day in the treatment of the human body, that physicians separate the soul from the body."[9] In *Evolution of the Brain, Creation of the Self*, physiologist and Nobel laureate Sir John Eccles strongly stated, "I maintain that the human mystery is incredibly demeaned by scientific reductionism ... We have to recognize that we are spiritual beings with souls existing in a spiritual world, as well as material beings with bodies and brains existing in a material world."[10]

But is modern medicine ready to acknowledge the role of spirituality in the pursuit of health and wellness? Apparently so. A 2010 study of medical schools found that 90 per cent offer courses on spirituality and health.[11] Flagship programs at George Washington University Medical School, Harvard Medical School and others explore concepts of spirituality as relevant and meaningful to wellbeing, not only for the patient but also for the practitioner.[12]

Tools and Skills for Expanded Perception

Over my years of teaching, I have noticed that medical intuition does not work better for one profession over another. A natural predisposition for intuition is also not a requirement. I have taught skeptics and true believers alike. Medical intuition can help wellness professionals do their jobs with greater discernment into the human condition. And certainly, we all have the ability to access intuition for our own wellbeing.

There are many ways in which medical intuitives gather information. Following are some fundamental components of the practice.

Life Force Energy: The Vital Spark

The belief in a vital life force energy that can influence and enhance our physical health has been a part of recorded history for thousands of years.

Ayurveda, a 5,000-year-old system of medicine from India, defines this vital force as *prana*, a Sanskrit term meaning "exhalation" or "breath of life." The ancient Greeks theorized vital life force as *pneuma*, the connection between "breath" and the soul or spirit. Traditional Chinese Medicine (TCM), which dates back to the third century BCE, embodies this energy as *qi* (*chi*), meaning "air," or "breath." The movement of *qi* through a system of meridians, or channels in the body, is considered basic to human health.

From the 1600s, early founders of modern chemistry, biology and physiology defined the idea of a "vital spark" of life force as "vitalism" – the belief that "living organisms are fundamentally different from non-living entities because they contain some non-physical element or are governed by different principles than are inanimate things."[13] This non-physical element was thought to be a distinctive spirit or substance that infused all living beings.

Vitalism was founded on the holistic principles of the body's natural healing ability, the role of healer as facilitator, and the influence of the mind on physical health. Prominent throughout the 18th and 19th centuries, vitalism stood in opposition to a growing concept that symptoms and diseases have a purely mechanistic and materialistic cause – what we know today as "biomedicine" or conventional, Western or allopathic medicine.

Both chiropractic medicine and osteopathy, founded in the late 1800s, are built on the philosophies of vitalism. Naturopathic doctors are still taught the foundations of vitalism, and it is considered an integral tenet of the practice.[14]

Contemporary energy healing methods, based on the rebalancing and restoration of vital life force energy, now use the term "subtle energy." But, regardless of the name, people have long understood that there is an intangible form of energy that imbues, engages and animates all life.

The Biofield

Paracelsus, a 16th-century Swiss alchemist and physician, reported "a healing energy that radiates within and around man like a luminous sphere."[15]

In 1992, a panel of researchers and alternative healing arts practitioners at the National Institutes of Health (NIH) chose the word "biofield" to describe a field of energy and information that surrounds, permeates and influences the human body.[16]

The biofield can be understood as containing both dense energy, similar to the electromagnetic fields generated by the heart and brain – as measured by electroencephalograms and electrocardiograms – and extremely subtle energy fields utilized in energy healing practices. Scientists are investigating the biofield to better understand its properties and functions, and theoretical foundations are still evolving.[17]

A study was launched in 2015 with the aim of directly observing the biofield through the phenomenon of the "phantom leaf effect."[18] Scientists used Kirlian photography, a technique that exposes an object to an electromagnetic field, capturing a luminescent aura-like glow surrounding and radiating from it.

Researchers severed 137 plant leaves and photographed each cut leaf. Of the severed leaves, 70 per cent showed the glowing corona of the entire leaf in detail, as if each cut leaf were still whole and intact. Though the results were quite controversial, scientists speculate that this phantom effect might show visual evidence of the biofield.

Also known as the "human energy field," the biofield consists of the chakra system and the aura, or auric field.[19] The auric field is described as multiple layers of energy that surround the body. Medical intuitives may perceive the aura as a series of colors, energy fields, vibrations or frequencies.

The chakra system is derived from the ancient Hindu philosophy of spiritual energy centers contained within the human body. Roughly aligned with the glands of the endocrine system, six major chakras are positioned along the spine, with a seventh chakra situated at the top of the head. Chakras are depicted in the sequential colors of the rainbow and as the unfolding petals of a lotus flower. Each chakra governs an aspect of human awareness: physical security, emotional balance, self-identity, love, communication, intuition and the higher spiritual states of consciousness. The chakras also relate to various organs and body systems.

A medical intuitive can review disturbances and blockages in the flow of energy within the biofield. If one pulls apart the schematic of how an illness may develop, subtle energy changes can be intuitively observed early in the process. A person may sense that something is "off," but may not be able to identify what it might be. Trained medical intuitives may recognize anomalies or disruptions in a client's biofield before an issue manifests, and can then refer the client to their licensed healthcare provider.

The Physical Body

Many people ask me if a medical education is needed to become a medical intuitive. Although wellness professionals come from a broad range of knowledge and practice, I consider a basic working knowledge of the major body systems to be a requirement for the skill.

C. Norman Shealy, a neurosurgeon and pioneering advocate of medical intuition, stated, "Medical intuition ... to be useful from a medical point of view ... requires that you know the physical location of a medically diagnosable problem as well as at least the physiological (electrical/chemical) 'cause' of the problem."[20]

The Meta-Senses

Medical intuitives access information with their meta-senses. "Meta" means "beyond," or an expanded experience of our five traditional senses. Also known as the *clairs*, a French word meaning "clear," some of the more well-known meta-senses are claircognizance or "clear knowing," clairsentience or "clear feeling," clairaudience or "clear hearing," and clairvoyance or "clear seeing" (*see* more in Chapter 8).

Medical intuitives use a variety of advanced meta-senses. A 2021 survey of professional medical intuitives found that claircognizance was the most used meta-sense at 39 per cent, followed by clairvoyance at 31 per cent and clairsentience at 22 per cent.[21] The primary meta-sense I practice is clairvoyance, or "mind's eye" intuition. I have found that pinpoint clairvoyant scanning allows me to view images of the anatomy, physiology and biofield in great detail.

Our Life Story

I consider everyone's history to be their own hero's journey of exploration, adversity and transformation. The kaleidoscope of our lives tells the story of our bodies, minds and spirits.

Western medicine is beginning to catch on. Narrative-based medicine was developed to help doctors shift from purely problem-solving to listening to their patients' stories of illness with empathy and understanding.[22] Not surprisingly, this approach has been found to strengthen the doctor–patient relationship and improve patient health outcomes. The bottom line is that people have an essential need to be heard and understood by their healthcare providers. And our own bodies have a deep need to be heard, as well.

We may have a memory of when a health issue began, and our medical records may corroborate it, but our bodies and biofields may have a completely different story to tell. By honing in on pivotal moments in a person's life history, medical intuition can reveal when and where an imbalance may have originally begun, why it may have occurred and how it might shift.

This intuitive viewpoint can offer a complete narrative that includes our beliefs, thoughts and emotions, and how we process and integrate our life experiences. Accessing this profound storyline is one of the great gifts of medical intuition as it can bring together seemingly disparate information into a cohesive whole.

Although you may be familiar with the concepts of intuition, you may also be asking, "How does a medical intuitive actually do this?" I will start with a memorable case study that illustrates these elements. When wellness professionals hear this account, even the most skeptical are intrigued by the potential of medical intuition.

CASE STUDY: CLAUDIA

An accomplished businesswoman in her mid-forties, Claudia came to see me with a persistent case of tendinitis in her wrist, which had been troubling her for about a month. She had seen her doctor and her acupuncturist, but nothing she had tried was working. Claudia wasn't aware of any obvious reasons for the flare-up, and tendinitis wasn't a chronic issue for her. In her words, it showed up "out of the blue."

With the meta-sense of clairvoyance, I used my medical intuitive skills to take a look. Her tendons looked inflamed and painful. Directly underneath the tendons, I observed a healed fracture in the bones of her wrist. In Claudia's biofield, I also perceived the energy of emotional pain and grief, which hovered like a dark cloud around the area.

I asked her wrist to show me where the tendinitis began. In my mind's eye, I saw her in her early twenties, playing tennis with her boyfriend. In an instant, she tripped and fell, fracturing her wrist exactly where I had detected the bone scar. The next defining moment showed Claudia in a hospital Emergency Room. As her injury was being treated, her boyfriend chose that very moment to break up with her. There it was. Claudia's wrist had stored not only the intense physical trauma of the fracture, but also the shock and emotional pain of the unexpected and sudden break-up.

When I explained what I saw, Claudia confirmed the incident and was quiet for a moment. She then said that her recent partner of ten years had broken up with her a month earlier, just before the tendinitis appeared. The emotional pain she was dealing with in the present had activated the stuck, unresolved grief and pain from her past. In Claudia's case, this combination of past and present trauma had manifested in severe tendinitis.

However, her wrist wasn't finished showing me images from her life. I then saw her at five years old, huddled in a dark closet. A woman was hitting her repeatedly with a cane. Little Claudia had her arm raised for protection. The cane was landing blows directly in the same spot where she had broken her wrist in her twenties, and where the tendinitis was now causing pain.

Claudia confirmed that her mentally ill mother used to beat her with a cane and lock her in a dark hallway closet. Claudia's wrist was holding on to a lifetime of emotional pain, physical trauma and grief.

Although she had memories of these specific life events, Claudia would never have put those puzzle pieces together to understand why tendinitis had flared up in the present. Logically, it didn't make sense, but her body had its own point of view. Claudia's wrist indicated that her unresolved emotions were the primary issue holding back its ability to heal fully.

I checked in with Claudia a few days later. She told me that the pain in her wrist had completely gone. She also said she felt calmer and more focused, and was finally able to begin processing the distress of her recent break-up. By simply hearing what her wrist had to tell her, Claudia's body and emotions were able to find balance.

Claudia's story is a perfect example of how much information the body holds and what it can tell us, when given the opportunity. This case study also demonstrates how I use a deliberate method of intuitive inquiry to gain answers directly from the body's own wisdom and unique perspective. We are not a collection of body parts and isolated events. Our entire experience of life, our emotions and our thoughts have a direct impact on our health and wellbeing.

EXERCISE: AM I INTUITIVE?

Can you remember a moment from your childhood when you had a strong intuition? What did it feel like? Did you tell anyone about it? How did they react?

Have you noticed any interesting coincidences in your daily life, such as a friend calling or emailing you just moments after you had thought about them? Have you ever found the perfect parking place by mentally asking to be guided to it by "The Parking Spot Angel"? Can you think of occasions when you just *knew* something was about to happen … and it did?

Journal Practice: In an intuition journal, begin to keep track of when intuitive incidents like this occur. Acknowledging your natural intuition and personal intuitive style can help you to grow and develop it.

CHAPTER 2
WHAT IS MEDICAL INTUITION?

Intuition is the clear conception of the whole at once.

Johann Kaspar Lavater

Before I define what medical intuition is, it's important to understand what it is not. Although medical intuition uses the term "medical," it is not the practice of medicine, psychotherapy or any other licensed healthcare practice. Medical intuition is not a substitute or replacement for medical or psychological advice or diagnosis.

The foundational skill of a medical intuitive assessment, also known as "scanning" or "reading," is not a treatment, intervention or any direct healing method in itself. Medical intuition is not intended to affect, manipulate or influence a client or patient's physical body, biofield or emotional state. Medical intuition is not the practice of health or lifestyle coaching, counseling, hypnotherapy, energy healing or any other alternative healing arts method.

And finally, although practitioners may feel it deepens their personal concepts of spirituality, medical intuition does not require any specific philosophy, religious or spiritual affiliation.

A New Definition of Medical Intuition
In 2005, the Institute of Medicine (IOM) convened a committee of experts to study the use of complementary and alternative medicine in the United States.[1] Their report defined medical

intuition as, "the utilization of a focused, intuitive instinct to 'diagnose' or 'read' energetic and frequency information in and around the human body." With all due respect to the IOM experts, the word "diagnose" is not used correctly in their definition. A diagnosis implies a sequential process of analysis through evaluation of medical history, physical examination and testing. Only a licensed medical professional can provide a diagnosis. Holistic psychiatrist, author and researcher Daniel Benor suggested the more accurate term "intuitive assessment" for medical intuition.[2]

The basis of medical intuition is that the body and the biofield hold information pertaining not only to physical imbalance, but also to emotional, mental and spiritual imbalances.

Medical intuition is designed to bring the underlying energetic causes and drivers of illness, imbalance and disease to conscious awareness, to help promote wellbeing in body, mind and spirit. As you will discover, this invaluable skill is intended to provide a comprehensive, whole-person context for health.

Here is a new definition of medical intuition:

- Medical intuition is a skill of intuitive observation and assessment using a system of expanded perception gained through the development of the human sense of intuition.
- Medical intuition focuses on in-depth intuitive scanning designed to obtain information from both the physical body systems and the biofield.
- Medical intuition is intended to identify and assess energetic patterns in both the physical body systems and the biofield that may correspond to illness, imbalance and disease.
- Medical intuition is designed to address the energetic influence of thoughts, beliefs and emotions, and how they may impact the health and wellbeing of an individual.

We are deeply interested in knowing what our bodies really want for optimal health and balance. Medical intuition offers clients the potential to gain greater personal awareness and insight, and to become a partner in their own wellness journey.

For the healthcare professional, medical intuition offers the opportunity to deliver fast, pertinent intuitive health assessments for a cost-effective, targeted approach to a patient or client's concerns. Most importantly, medical intuition can help unlock the door to relevant and profound breakthroughs when people aren't healing, despite best efforts.

Changing Times, Changing Terms

This is a time of rapid change in healthcare. Concepts are shifting as the public accepts modalities across a wide spectrum of wellness options. So, where does medical intuition fit into this swiftly changing landscape?

Currently, medical intuition is not a licensed profession in the United States and falls under the canopy of Complementary and Alternative Medicine (CAM). CAM is a consensus term for medical and health systems, practices and products that are not presently part of standard conventional medicine.[3]

In 2014, the US National Institutes of Health (NIH) replaced the term "Complementary and Alternative Medicine" with "Complementary and Integrative Health" (CIH) at the federal level. The NIH defines integrative health as "a holistic, patient-focused approach to health care and wellness."[4] To help settle confusion over the terms, the NIH defined "alternative" as non-mainstream healthcare practices used *in place of* conventional medicine, and "complementary" as non-mainstream practices used *together with* conventional medicine. Medical intuition can be used in both of these ways – as a standalone alternative practice and as a complementary and integrative practice.

Although these terms are evolving, US state laws referring to CAM have not yet changed. As medical intuitive practitioners come from a wide variety of backgrounds, they must be aware of their legally defined scope of practice, including local, state and federal laws governing healthcare providers.

Where Is the New Research?

There is much published research on the general use of intuition in healthcare. However, the research focused solely on the skill of medical intuition is extremely limited. As of this writing, only a relatively small number of studies have been published, almost all of which were conducted at least 20 years ago. Though this was disheartening to learn, it also became glaringly obvious to me that it was time for new peer-reviewed research of all kinds – qualitative, quantitative and case studies.

In late 2018, I launched a pilot study with the support of Paul J. Mills, Professor of Family Medicine and Public Health, Director of the Center of Excellence for Research and Training in Integrative Health at the University of California, San Diego, and Director of Research for the Chopra Foundation. The study focused on trained medical intuitives' accuracy rates for perceiving physical complaints, potential root causes and relevant life history.[5]

Remarkable Results from a Blinded Study

Five certified graduates of my training program served as the study's practitioners, along with 67 volunteer subjects. None of the subjects' health or medical history was given to the medical intuitives.

After their sessions, the subjects filled out an anonymous survey. We were thrilled with the results. The subjects rated the medical intuitives as 94 per cent accurate in locating and evaluating their main physical issues, and 98 per cent accurate in intuiting specific events from their lives that related to their health issues. About half of the subjects had received a diagnosis from their doctor for their health issue. It was exciting to see that the subjects rated the medical intuitives' evaluations as 94 per cent consistent with their known diagnoses. (To reiterate, the medical intuitives did not diagnose, but described the intuited information only.) These outstanding findings support the ideal scenario for medical intuitives as valued members of the healthcare team (*see* more in Chapter 5).

The survey also included questions on what the subjects thought of medical intuition as a support to their own health and wellness care. They were extremely positive and receptive, with an overall satisfaction level of 99 per cent, and 97 per cent indicated they would recommend medical intuition to others. Needless to say, these outcomes were both gratifying and validating. A complete review of the research is included in Chapter 4.

The study, "Assessing the Accuracy of Medical Intuition: A Subjective and Exploratory Study," was published in the *Journal of Alternative and Complementary Medicine (JACM)* in November 2020. It was co-authored by Dr. Mills, whose generous efforts have been integral in supporting this research.

The article achieved high-impact status (extensive readership and citations) at *JACM*, which attests to the growing interest in this emerging field. The findings have also been featured at leading integrative health organizations, including the Academy of Integrative Health & Medicine (AIHM), the American Holistic Nurses Association (AHNA), the Andrew Weil Center for Integrative Medicine at the University of Arizona, the Integrative Health Policy Consortium (IHPC), and the International Congress on Integrative Medicine & Health (ICIMH).

Who Uses Medical Intuition in their Wellness Practice?

The diversity of wellness professionals who use medical intuition might surprise you. In 2020, a survey was distributed to self-identified medical intuitives in the US.[6] Among those surveyed, 82 per cent report they assist licensed healthcare providers with medical intuition:

- 22 per cent assist physicians and specialists, such as primary care practitioners, osteopathic doctors, pediatricians, cardiologists and others

- 21 per cent assist other medical providers, such as physician assistants, nurse practitioners, naturopathic doctors, nurses, and allied healthcare professionals
- 21 per cent assist mental healthcare providers, such as psychologists, psychiatrists, licensed social workers and therapists
- 18 per cent assist licensed CIH providers, such as acupuncturists, chiropractors and licensed massage therapists.

Additionally, 86 per cent receive referrals for medical intuitive services from licensed healthcare providers:

- 19 per cent from physicians and specialists
- 23 per cent from other medical providers
- 26 per cent from mental healthcare providers
- 18 per cent from CIH providers.

Would you also be impressed to learn that 30 per cent of professional medical intuitives surveyed are licensed healthcare providers themselves? These unprecedented results show that medical intuition is being used more widely throughout healthcare than anyone had anticipated.

The Elephant in the Exam Room

In Chapter 1, I mentioned my conversations with doctors who consult with medical intuitives. Our talks invariably lead to a deeper discussion about the many pitfalls, headaches and heartaches inherent in the current medical system. My eyes have been opened to the stresses they regularly deal with, including significantly less one-on-one time with their patients and an ever-growing mountain of daily paperwork. Though medical intuition can't help with administrative duties, it is uniquely equipped to assist with some of the biggest challenges doctors may face. Let me explain.

Medical error is a major concern for patients and doctors. It is, quite honestly, the "elephant" in the clinic and hospital room. The term covers a range of issues, including diagnostic error, drug injury, undertreatment, overtreatment, not ordering needed tests and not addressing atypical findings.[7] A sobering report in the *BMJ* shows US deaths from medical error at 250,000 per year, making it the third leading cause of death after heart disease and cancer.[8] Some studies estimate deaths from medical error at 400,000 annually – a staggering statistic.[9]

According to another study in the *BMJ*, 10–15 per cent of diagnoses are incorrect, including missed primary or differential diagnoses, and wrong or delayed diagnoses.[10] It should be no surprise that diagnostic error regularly tops the list in patient worries.[11] Adding to this, excessive testing and overtreatment can cause harm, physically, emotionally and financially. Estimated at a cost of more than $200 billion annually, overtreatment accounts for up to one-third of all healthcare spending in the US.[12] Physicians themselves estimate that more than 20 per cent of prescriptions, tests and procedures are unneeded.[13] All of this adds up to billions in preventable costs, worse patient outcomes, untold suffering, and even lost lives.

If you work in healthcare, you certainly know more about these challenges than I do. What I know is that medical intuition is ideally suited to help. In this book, you will find a vision for game-changing models of doctor *and* medical intuitive, and doctor *as* medical intuitive. You will read in practitioners' own words how medical intuition has optimized and enhanced their processes by helping them to:

- save time with fast, pertinent information
- optimize wellness assessments and evaluations
- reduce costs with a targeted plan for integrative care options
- support compliance by providing insight and awareness
- promote useful preventive care
- discover the underlying causes of physical, emotional and environmental factors

- provide a comprehensive approach for body, mind and spirit wellbeing.

This reality is not waiting in some misty, far-off future. It is available right now. And many experts agree:

> *Being a physician who is also a medical intuitive, I can intervene before symptoms manifest and work toward a preventive treatment. That is the whole strategy for catching issues early. And, that is the reason we do so many screening tests, though none of them are really that definitive. If you have assurance that you could test something specific very early, that is a game-changer in medicine.*
>
> Lloyd Costello, MD

> *Having trained medical intuitives in the biomedical setting, particularly in emergency departments where time for proper treatment is crucial, could make significant contributions to improve the health of many patients.*
>
> Paul J. Mills, PhD, Professor and Chief of Family Medicine, University of California San Diego School of Medicine

> *Medical intuition can help with patients who have difficult cases or illnesses of a multifactorial nature. It can provide a unique insight into the problem including its underlying energetic and mind–body factors. It also engages the patient in their own healing process by lifting the veil on the causes of deep-rooted patterns stemming from unconscious energetic constructs. As medical professionals, we can offer this service to our patients directly via our enhanced intuitive and diagnostic abilities, or by hiring a qualified medical intuitive in our practice.*
>
> Maria Gentile, DO, CMIP

As a doctor, I believe it would be incredibly valuable to have a patient seen by a certified medical intuitive to help me determine which tests would be most useful. The cost savings in healthcare could be significant.

Larry Burk, MD, CEHP,
holistic radiologist and author

Medical intuition is a practical and testable phenomenon. If people really knew about medical intuition, it would change our healthcare system. However, the whole structure of the current medical model doesn't allow space for this. I feel that a shift to integrate intuition is going to come organically from the "bottom up," with practitioners incorporating it into their practice as they learn its usefulness, and patients demanding it when they see how it benefits them.

Helané Wahbeh, ND, MCR, Director of
Research, Institute of Noetic Sciences (IONS)

Medical intuition is the future of global healthcare. It is a learnable way of accessing information to not only gain insight into the etiology of the disease process but also to determine what may lead to optimal health and wellness. It is the missing piece in the Western medical model that has the potential to fast-track healing.

Karandeep Singh, MD

Overcoming Bias: "This" Does Not Always Equal "That"

There is another pitfall that medical intuition is expressly designed to address – one that is pervasive yet is almost completely overlooked, and exists in every area of healthcare – the problem of practitioner "bias."[14]

Let me be clear from the start that I am not a proponent of one mode of healthcare over another. In a medical intuitive assessment, the practitioner's preferences or biases on health choices should *never* enter into the process. This may seem odd, but it is a fundamental principle of medical intuition.

Why is a lack of bias so important? In my career I have never seen a one-size-fits-all basis for wellness. A bias can act as a blinder to finding the best possible pathways to health. The truth is, we need every kind of care available, from the life-saving drugs, procedures and technologies of conventional medicine, to the best of complementary and alternative health disciplines. Most of all, we need a healthcare system that works.

Confirmation bias, also called cognitive bias, is the tendency to look only for evidence that confirms our preexisting ideas and beliefs. According to a review of 35 years of research on clinical decision-making, cognitive biases were associated with diagnostic inaccuracies in up to 77 per cent of cases.[15] Biases create overconfidence, low risk tolerance, anchoring to a single piece of information, and wishful thinking, which leads to overestimating rewards and underestimating risks.

Holistic practices, including energy-based healing methods, can also suffer from the same tunnel-vision thinking. Whether the assertion is from mainstream medicine that *this* set of symptoms must correlate to *that* illness, or from the holistic standpoint that *this* energetic information must correspond to *that* wellness issue – these fixed positions can turn guidelines into hard lines.

In contrast, medical intuition offers the absence of bias by tapping directly into the body's own perspective. From here, we can gain information that is unfiltered by our own limiting beliefs or concepts, or even by our personal body of knowledge.

Of course, we expect a specialist to be an expert in their field, and so we should. But a standardized approach can be deeply frustrating for people who have not found a clear path to wellness. They may feel their healthcare providers are not listening to or understanding them, which can affect compliance and may even allow health problems to go untreated for years.[16] And what about those with chronic symptoms but normal lab results, or with conditions that don't fit the current modes of care, such as

Lyme disease, environmental sensitivities and leaky gut, among others? At a time when people may be at their most vulnerable, they can end up feeling betrayed, disillusioned or hopeless.

Our healthcare providers are also suffering. The doctors and nurses in my classes tell me about their burnout from overwork, unrelenting job stress, and compassion fatigue.[17] The pressures of an overburdened medical system are taking a heavy toll on medical providers' physical and emotional health.

How Can Medical Intuition Help?

The statistics on medical errors, extreme medical costs and un-happy patients and practitioners are truly shocking. It is time to change this paradigm. The following are just a few examples from healthcare professionals on how medical intuition has transformed their practices.

Medical intuition was a game-changer for me. I'm able to get to the root of my patients' issues without wasting precious time and unnecessary expense. My patients have expressed their gratitude for how much it has helped them. One of the greatest rewards is to be able to help another human being when others are unable.
Marie Mendoza-Cipollo, DC, CMIP, HC

Adding medical intuition to my acupuncture practice helped me more accurately diagnose my patients, particularly with complex and difficult cases where there are multiple imbalances compounding each other. Medical intuition is invaluable in dissecting and parceling out the complexities and honing in on the root cause, or causes, of disease.
Holly Scalmanini, LAc

Medical intuition provides a matrix through which all of my holistic healing and medical knowledge can be processed and understood. The medical intuitive process helps to identify core issues at the root of my patients' health issues, and this awareness can contribute to true healing on a very deep level.

Christine Allison, RN, BSN, CMIP

Medical intuition allows me to see "qi" in action. As a medical intuitive, I can see the physical/emotional pattern of a bodily dysfunction, and give useful recommendations on options. These are powerful, analytical and creative tools for health.

Natasha Reiss, LAc, MSTOM, CMIP

As a licensed clinical psychologist, I am able to "see" where the energy is blocked at the origins of my clients' issues. I'm getting great feedback from my clients about sudden transformations in their lives.

Diane Puchbauer, PsyD

As a holistic nurse, medical intuition gives me tools to sharpen my assessment skills and offer a deeper level of understanding. I now have an expanded awareness of how to use my intuition to help guide people toward whole-person care and new opportunities for increased wellness. Medical intuition brought the values of holistic nursing into focus.

Sandy Robertson, RN, MSN,
HNB-BC, CHTP, CMIP

What to Expect When Working with a Medical Intuitive

As I mentioned in the previous chapter, medical intuitives use advanced meta-sensory skills, such as intuitive *seeing, feeling, hearing* or *knowing*, also known as the *clairs*. They may use one meta-sense exclusively or a blend of several at a time.

My preferred method is clairvoyance, or *seeing* in the mind's eye. I intuitively see highly detailed visuals of the anatomy and physiology, at rest or in action, down to the cellular level. I may see symbolic, exaggerated or abstract imagery. I may see the body in realistic color, or as a series of colors.

The aura and chakra system are filled with vital insights that can relate to the emotional, mental or spiritual aspects of a wellness issue. During a session, I can look for energetic disturbances that may be limiting or blocking the natural flow of energy. I may also review specific scenes from a client's life history. These "mental movies" are rich with information, which can help the client become aware of the intrinsic connections between the events of their lives and their health. Finally, medical intuition can support the client in navigating wellness options by interacting directly with their body's own wisdom.

I never assume that what I see in one client's energy, for example a particular symbol or color, will mean the same thing in every client's energy. Doing so would be using a pre-existing bias or belief that would hinder my ability to see clearly. Instead, my job is to assess the energetic information that is unique to each individual and their own physical and energetic systems.

This is not a random or chaotic technique. I call it being an "intuitive detective" – a deliberate, step-by-step process of intuitive investigation. Each cell, organ and system has its own innate consciousness and can express itself in meaningful ways. The biofield can be described as a "filing cabinet" filled with a wealth of information. A qualified medical intuitive can access the energetic details of past and present issues. Because this material is so personal and varied, medical intuition holds significant possibilities for healthcare.

One hallmark of medical intuition is the ability to perform an accurate assessment without having any prior knowledge of a person's health issues or life history. Sessions can also be performed remotely for clients all over the world, by telephone or internet. In fact, a client does not even need to be in the present moment with a medical intuitive while a session is in progress.

This last point brings up some very important ethical considerations. Practitioner ethics, scope of practice and legal risk factors must be understood. Without strong standards and competent training, medical intuition will not be able to progress.

An excellent guide to establishing an ethical and legally sound practice is *Practice Energy Healing in Integrity: The Joy of Offering Your Gifts Legally and Ethically*, written by Midge Murphy, a legal risk consultant who is also an energy healing practitioner.[18] Attorney Michael H. Cohen's book, *Future Medicine*, is another outstanding resource.[19]

There are spiritual ethics to consider as well. As medical intuition accesses broader levels of consciousness, practitioners must be mindful to not blur ethical lines. This includes being vigilant to not project their own beliefs or biases, or overstep the power differential. The power differential is the authority a practitioner is granted by a client – a dynamic that can be amplified when using intuitive skills. It is crucial that a medical intuitive creates an ethical and respectful atmosphere.

There are many facets to this subject. Here are some points to be aware of when choosing a medical intuitive to work with.

A professional medical intuitive:

- complies with local, state and federal laws
- offers safe and professional practices
- operates only within their legally defined scope of practice
- does not diagnose or prescribe unless legally licensed to do so
- maintains the client's rights to privacy and confidentiality
- does not make medical claims or promises
- is respectful of the power differential between practitioner and client
- establishes clear and appropriate boundaries
- receives the client's informed consent prior to a session
- refers the client to a licensed healthcare provider for medical or psychological care

- explains costs, policies and the nature of their services in advance
- and, above all, honors the free will of the client.

The Medical Intuitive Assessment

"Can you take a 'look' at one of my patients? Nothing seems to be working." This question was becoming more and more common. It seemed that I had developed an under-the-radar reputation with some of the local physicians. Despite the fact that my business card said "Energy Healing Practitioner," they increasingly contacted me for intuitive assessments only. They were not at all interested in energy healing. I eventually changed my business card to read, "Medical Intuitive."

Early in my career, I realized the power of the intuitive assessment for the value and level of detail it brought to these doctors. I began to develop my most valuable service – the Medical Intuitive Assessment. This efficient, streamlined method has allowed me to formalize and teach the practical application of medical intuition.

Many medical intuitives use their intuition in combination with an energy healing modality. In my practice, however, I have found medical intuition to be most effective as a separate assessment, used apart from energy healing. The case studies throughout this book are examples of this standalone approach.

Why not combine medical intuition with energy healing skills? The answer is not complex, but it is vital. In my energy healing work, I noticed that some clients would return with the same issue over and over, unable to release it. I wondered why some had deep healing experiences during or after a session, while others did not, even though I used my skills in the same way every time. I began to offer a medical intuitive assessment before, or in place of, an energy healing session. My goal was to intuitively *view* the reasons why an issue had manifested in the first place, and to find out why it was staying stuck. I was curious to know if this information would make a difference.

The messages in these sessions offered profound realizations for my clients. Again and again, they confirmed that the intuitive assessment was a key factor in helping them turn the corner in their health journey. After a while, it seemed silly for me to assume that my energy healing modality was needed before I'd first had a chance to ask the client's body and biofield what it actually wanted. This awareness fundamentally changed my practice forever.

Who May Need a Medical Intuitive?

Consider for a moment what kind of people may typically want to see a medical intuitive:

- People who have seen dozens of doctors for health conditions for which conventional medicine has no effective answers
- People whose conditions are not well researched because of a lack of funding or interest by the medical community
- People who are confused or overwhelmed by the number of health options available
- People who just don't feel well even though tests are normal or inconclusive
- People who may feel abandoned or abused by the medical system
- People who want to understand the deeper meanings behind their health challenges

I have seen all of these kinds of clients in the course of more than 20 years in practice. Each one of them has helped me develop and grow my intuitive abilities. A turning point in my understanding of the importance of what medical intuition can offer came a few years into my professional practice, when I worked with a young woman named Annie.

CASE STUDY: ANNIE

Annie, a lovely, vivacious woman in her early twenties, had been actively pursuing her dreams and goals. By the time I saw her, she was crippled with bouts of pain in her mid-back area and struggling emotionally. After many tests, her doctors could not find a conclusive reason for her pain. Eventually, her symptoms were deemed psychosomatic. Annie had been prescribed antidepressants and opioids for pain management.

As a last resort, her parents reached out to me to set up a session. Almost immediately, Annie's left kidney showed me a tiny crystallized shard that had started to move slightly out of the kidney, but then embedded itself at the top of the ureter tube. It didn't seem to want to budge. The shard was very small, but Annie could certainly feel the effect of it. After so much rejection from her doctors, however, even she doubted what her body was so desperately trying to tell her.

As a medical intuitive, I ask the body what it wants and needs to find balance. I asked the kidney, "What if Annie could drink enough water so that her body could naturally pass the shard?" Her kidney's reply was extremely clear. It said, "Go see a surgeon." I asked again, and received the same answer.

As I am not a licensed medical professional, I do not diagnose, prescribe or give medical advice. But I always encourage a client to find a licensed professional that may be able to help. I quickly sketched my intuitive observations on a piece of paper and gave it to Annie. I urged her to find a specialist who would be willing to take a closer look.

I didn't find out what had happened to Annie until several years later. Her parents told me they had found an excellent surgeon who believed Annie and took her case.

A procedure to remove the kidney stone was a success, and she was finally out of pain. Unfortunately, the story did not end there. Tragically, she had become addicted to the opioids she was prescribed and died of an overdose.

This devastating, heartbreaking outcome should never have happened. What if she had gone to see a medical intuitive earlier? What if her doctors had the opportunity to consult with a medical intuitive when the tests were inconclusive? Perhaps Annie would still be alive today.

Annie's story stayed with me, and turned my ideas about medical intuition from a novel and interesting talent to a potentially life-saving ability. From that day on, I understood that medical intuition should have a place in modern healthcare. It became my mission to teach this paradigm-shifting skill.

How did medical intuition help? It was evident from the start of our session that Annie's quality of life was suffering. At the time, the diagnostics available were not sufficient enough to pick up such a small kidney stone. I was able to validate her experience by perceiving her kidney's messages. Moreover, my intuitive assessment gave her the knowledge and confidence to not give up. The surgeon she consulted after our session correctly diagnosed and treated her kidney stone. As a medical intuitive, I was an interpreter and an advocate for the very loud message radiating from her body.

CHAPTER 3

A BRIEF HISTORY OF MEDICAL INTUITION

Nature affords a universal means of healing and preserving men.

Franz Anton Mesmer

Franz Anton Mesmer (1734–1815), a German physician, believed that an invisible vital force flows throughout the human body and that illness results from blockages in the flow.[1] Mesmer described this natural force as a "magnetic fluid" and compared the interaction in the body to the sun and moon's gravitational pull on the tides. His healing system, known as "animal magnetism" or "mesmerism," was vaunted as a new method to treat diseases of every kind.

High-profile cases and sensational cures made him extremely popular with the public, but the medical establishment considered him to be a charlatan. Nevertheless, Mesmer's ideas influenced science and medicine for more than 70 years, and formed the basis of modern hypnotherapy, mind–body concepts and contemporary energy healing modalities.

Some of the first published reports on intuitive assessments for health can be credited to the physicians and scientists of the late 18th and 19th centuries who adopted and advanced Mesmer's unconventional methods. In their experiments, they found that some mesmerized patients, with no medical background or knowledge, exhibited extraordinary intuitive abilities to accurately perceive health conditions.

Amand-Marie-Jacques de Chastenet, the Marquis de Puységur (1751–1825), was a scholar and disciple of Mesmer and an imortant figure in the early history of mesmerism.[2] Puységur suggested that mesmerism was an induced state of artificial somnambulism, a sleep-like, half-awake trance. Puységur logged many cases of remarkable abilities in his patients. One of his most famous was a young peasant named Victor Race who, while in a deep somnambulistic state, could clairvoyantly evaluate his own physical disorders and specify corresponding remedies, and was able to do the same for others.[3]

French naturalist Joseph P. F. Deleuze (1753–1835) published several seminal works on mesmerism, which included cases of his own patients' skills in discerning health issues while mesmerized. In the interests of research, he also took patients to the professional somnambulists of Paris, who offered clairvoyant health sessions for a fee. His peers frowned on this kind of sensationalistic display, but Deleuze had a point to make. Of the Parisian somnambulists, he wrote, "I have seen them, after a quarter of an hour of concentration and of silence, divine the origin, the cause, and the stages of the diseases, determine the seat of the pains, discover what no physician could perceive, and describe with exactitude the character, the habits, and the inclinations of those who consult them."[4]

In a posthumously published memoir, Deleuze admitted that in his accounts he had downplayed and even omitted some of the data he'd collected on the astonishing successes of mesmerism, as he feared the medical world was not ready to accept it.[5]

Many similar cases were reported in France and across Europe.[6] Physician Alexandre J. F. Bertrand (1795–1831) conducted experiments with a mesmerized female patient and found that she could feel the physical symptoms and pain of others. She was even able to detect illnesses that Dr. Bertrand had missed.[7] In 1818, physiologist D. Velianski, a medical professor at the Imperial Academy of St. Petersburg, Russia, outlined the stages of the somnambulist's trance process, including the point at which a patient could identify their own physical ailment and a correct course of treatment.[8]

Although many physicians and scientists received these reports with great excitement, the medical societies regarded them with a good deal of skepticism, if not outright hostility. All of the incidents were subject to scrutiny, and commissions were convened to further examine the evidence.

Investigating Mesmerism

Based on the incredible claims of Mesmer, Puységur and others, in 1784 Louis XVI appointed the first commission to investigate the very existence of animal magnetism.[9] The French Royal Commission of Inquiry, which included Benjamin Franklin in his role as US Ambassador to France, found no proof for Mesmer's magnetic fluid and warned against it. But the practice had already captured the fascination of the public and the growing curiosity of scientists.

Over the next 42 years, more and more evidence of the astounding health benefits and clairvoyant wonders of mesmerism were published. A second commission was appointed in 1826 by the French Academies of the Sciences and of Medicine.[10] The commissioners, dubious about mesmeric "diagnosis," offered three patients as test subjects. To demonstrate, physician Dr. P. Foissac (1801–est. 1884) brought in a somnambulist named Celine. With no medical training or knowledge of the patients' conditions, she was able to correctly describe their maladies and give accurate treatment recommendations. For one patient being treated with mercury, she pointed out that the remedy was causing the patient's symptoms, rather than the illness itself. The doctors ignored her advice and the patient died soon after. An autopsy determined that Celine's perceptions had been correct.

The commissioners were duly impressed, though they had no explanation for the phenomena. Unanimously, they found reason to consider the practice valid and encouraged further research. In a report presented in 1831, they concluded that mesmerism resulted in "new faculties, which have been designated by the terms clairvoyance, intuition ... when this state cannot be ascribed to any other cause."[11] Finally, mesmerism, somnambulism, and the unique intuitive faculties they bestowed, were deemed to exist.

Unfortunately, it was not to last. The medical establishment doubled down on their opposition, and eventually mesmerism was roundly rejected in scientific circles.[12]

Even so, maverick practitioners continued their research, including John Elliotson (1791–1868), a prominent British physician who also promoted the first use of the stethoscope; physician James Esdaile (1808–1859), who employed mesmerism as a form of anesthesia; and surgeon James Braid (1795–1860), considered a pioneer of modern hypnotism.[13]

The Spiritualists

While the medical world had turned its back on mesmerism, clairvoyance and other intuitive marvels, the public remained steadfast in their enthusiasm. By the 1850s, the Spiritualist movement was in full swing.[14] In both the US and Europe, a craze for all things paranormal and an obsession with the afterlife were in vogue in much of cultured society. Consultations with spirit mediums were so popular that as many as eight séances were hosted by President Abraham Lincoln at the White House.[15]

Though it may be difficult for us to appreciate the fervor of the times, many of the era's greatest thinkers, including lauded physicians, philosophers, scientists and inventors, were ardent believers who supported rigorous research into paranormal claims. Two American medical intuitives identified with the Spiritualist movement are worth noting.

Andrew Jackson Davis (1826–1910), considered a founder of Spiritualism, was a colorful and controversial figure.[16] As a teenager he had a mesmerism session. While in a trance, Davis found he could see into the human body as if it were transparent.

Similar to the European clairvoyants, he was able to locate maladies and pinpoint cures. Known as the "Poughkeepsie Seer," Davis went on to produce some of Spiritualism's most influential writings.

Maria B. Hayden (1824–1883), a medium from Boston, Massachusetts, is primarily credited for bringing Spiritualism to England.[17] In her forties, she graduated from medical school – quite an accomplishment for a woman of her time. She gained a reputation for accurate medical diagnoses by holding the hand of a subject and intuiting their state of physical health, a practice she dubbed "clairsympathy." Dr. Hayden gained the respect of her colleagues as one of the nation's first "psychic" physicians.

The term "medical intuitive" would not be coined for another 100 years. However, the accomplishments of these early clairvoyant somnambulists and spiritualists distinguished them as the first recorded medical intuitives.

The 18th and 19th centuries were an exhilarating time for the scientific exploration of intuitive phenomena. Eventually, though, these bold ideas were overtaken by the mechanistic biomedical model and faded out in the early 20th century.[18] Fortunately, burgeoning research is once again exploring the integral aspects of intuition and human consciousness, and their roles in health and wellbeing.

Trailblazers of Medical Intuition

There are four Americans whose life's work can be recognized as building the framework for contemporary medical intuition in the US. Each of them has added invaluable contributions to the body of work that came before, and blazed a trail of their own for others to follow.

Phineas P. Quimby's "Mind Cure"

The trouble is in the mind, for the body is only the house for the mind to dwell in … Therefore, if your mind has

*been deceived by some invisible enemy into a belief, you
have put it into the form of a disease, with or without your
knowledge. By my theory or truth I come in contact with
your enemy and restore you to health and happiness.*

Phineas Parkhurst Quimby[19]

One of the first recorded practices of mind–body methods dates back to Phineas Parkhurst Quimby (1802–1866). Quimby is regarded as the founder of the New Thought movement, a philosophy based on the belief that the mind has the ability to heal the body.[20]

Born in Lebanon, New Hampshire, Quimby became a clockmaker. As a young man, he fell ill with tuberculosis.[21] The harsh medications his doctors prescribed only made him feel worse, and his health deteriorated. A friend who had healed himself by riding horseback encouraged Quimby to do the same. While driving his horse and cart at a fast gallop, Quimby noticed that the intensity and excitement of the ride dissipated his symptoms, and his feelings of health and strength returned. This sparked his investigation into the connection between the mind and the body, and led to the development of his "mind cure," which he credited as healing him of tuberculosis.

In 1838, Quimby attended a lecture by Charles Poyen, a French mesmerist. Intrigued, Quimby began studying this new skill and became quite proficient. Together with a somnambulist named Lucius Burkmar, he toured the country giving lectures and demonstrations of clairvoyant "diagnosis" to enthralled audiences.

Later, Quimby moved away from mesmerism to focus on his mind cure method. He believed that disease was caused by false beliefs and that all sickness originated in the mind. His techniques were based on correcting "errors" in thinking to help produce a physical healing effect. In 1859, Quimby began his healing practice in Portland, Maine, and treated more than 12,000 patients.[22]

Quimby's ideas inspired early New Thought leaders, including Norman Vincent Peale, Ernest Holmes and psychologist William James, known as the founder of positive psychology.

Edgar Cayce: Medical Clairvoyant

Know that all healing forces are within, not without! The applications from without are merely to create within a coordinating mental and spiritual force.

Edgar Cayce[23]

Much has been documented about the work of the enigmatic Edgar Cayce (1877–1945).[24] As a highly intuitive child in Hopkinsville, Kentucky, he reported speaking with dead relatives and spirits from other realms. In school Cayce displayed an extraordinary ability to learn his lessons by taking a short nap on a book and waking up with the contents fully memorized. Cayce later developed his distinctive technique of using a self-induced sleep-trance state to receive intuitive information for physical ailments and holistic-based remedies.

In 1928, Cayce opened his hospital in Virginia Beach, Virginia.[25] His clinic dealt almost exclusively with healing the digestive system and conditions that prevented the "proper equilibrium of the assimilating system."[26] Today, we understand gut health as critical to the functioning of the immune system, brain health and whole-body balance. Cayce's intuitions are now supported by extensive research and are foundational to the principles of integrative healthcare.[27] Due to the Great Depression, the hospital venture was short-lived. In 1931, the Association for Research and Enlightenment (A.R.E.) center was founded to carry on his work.

Cayce can also be credited with creating one of the first natural pharmacopeias.[28] His hospital documented his findings and built a vast compendium of holistic health interventions. These included osteopathy, colonics, homeopathy, essential oils, magnets, massage and much more – many of which are now well established and evidence-supported. Though much of Cayce's writings focused on spiritual topics, his work as a medical clairvoyant was well ahead of his time.

Caroline Myss & C. Norman Shealy: Medical Intuition Innovators

Your biography becomes your biology.

Caroline Myss[29]

One of the most respected names in the field of medical intuition is author, speaker and teacher Caroline Myss. Her book, *Anatomy of the Spirit*, introduced medical intuition to the world and influenced a generation of intuitives.[30] Appearances on *The Oprah Winfrey Show* established her as the premier authority on medical intuition.[31] Myss's books on healing and personal development continue to top the bestseller lists.

In 1985, Myss began a long-term collaboration with Dr. C. Norman Shealy, a Harvard-trained neurosurgeon, founding president of the American Holistic Medical Association, and a respected pioneer of chronic pain reduction methods.

Prior to meeting Myss, Dr. Shealy had worked with several medical intuitives to conduct his own studies (*see* Chapter 4). Dr. Shealy provided Myss with only a patient's name and age. She clairvoyantly "entered" the patient's body to examine their physical organs and systems, ascertaining their health issues and zeroing in on any emotional factors that may have contributed to their illness.[32] Dr. Shealy found Myss to be 93 per cent accurate.

Unsatisfied with the terms "clairvoyant" or "psychic," Dr. Shealy and Myss wanted to find an appropriate name for her unique process.[33] They created the term "medical intuitive" in 1988 based on concepts cultivated by the mesmerists of the 19th century. The name stuck and has been in use for over 30 years.

Intuition Influencers

In recent decades, there has been a resurgence of interest in medical intuition. Articles have appeared in *Medical Economics*, WebMD, *Townsend Letter*, Today's Practitioner, Gwyneth Paltrow's *Goop* and even in *Good Housekeeping* magazine.[34] Medical intuitives have been featured on *The Oprah Winfrey Show*, *The Doctors* and *The Dr. Oz Show*.[35] Other contemporary field leaders include psychiatrist Judith Orloff and neuropsychiatrist Mona Lisa Schulz.[36] And there are, of course, many talented and dedicated medical intuitives working quietly behind the scenes and out of the spotlight.

History shows us that the medical establishment has had difficulty accepting proof of intuition. Even so, forward-thinking doctors and researchers are open to the possibilities that medical intuition can offer. In the next chapter, you will read about the current scientific thought on intuition in healthcare.

CHAPTER 4

SHOW ME THE EVIDENCE: INTUITION IN HEALTHCARE

It is by logic that we prove, but by intuition that we discover.
Henri Poincaré

Logic, organization and order are at the very heart of scientific thought. Analytical thinking is what our minds do extremely well as we try to make sense of disparate or contradictory information. Evidence-based research that pushes the boundaries of convention creates new breakthrough systems that help humanity progress.

In an attempt to determine the facts from the fakes, scientific minds have sought to organize and catalog the mysteries of intuition within the rigors of the scientific method. Decades of research have led to compelling new approaches and realizations.[1]

People often argue that intuition doesn't work that way. It's random and unpredictable. It can't be contained, quantified or organized. But, as you will see, research shows that skilled medical intuitives can reproduce results consciously and deliberately at will, making intuition both accessible and reliable. In this chapter, I unpack some of the studies on intuition in the clinical setting and take a deep dive into the existing research on medical intuition.

The Clinical Hunch

Healthcare professionals recognize the importance of a "gut feeling" or a "hunch." A growing wealth of scientific literature acknowledges non-analytical reasoning as integral to clinical decision-making.[2] In fact, the Library of Medicine at the National Institutes of Health (NIH) is stocked with thousands of studies on how, when and why clinicians use their intuition.

Physician Trisha Greenhalgh is Professor of Primary Care Health Sciences at the University of Oxford, UK. She argues that intuitive insights are commonplace in general practice and should be accepted.[3] "Intuition is not unscientific," she writes. "It is a highly creative process, fundamental to hypothesis generation in science. The experienced practitioner should generate and follow clinical hunches, as well as (not instead of) applying the deductive principles of evidence-based medicine."

Professor Tim Mickleborough of the Ontario Institute for Studies in Education agrees.[4] "Technical knowledge alone is not sufficient to solve the complex problems that professionals face on a daily basis, and intuition … is crucial for any professional's practice," he writes.

How do doctors use their intuition? To find out, one study investigated real cases of physician intuition.[5] Eighteen family medicine doctors were interviewed about their intuitive decision-making processes with patients. Their responses were sorted into three different types of intuitions: "gut feelings," which triggered a sense of alarm that spurred them to take action; "recognitions," decisions made in the face of conflicting information or a lack of evidence; and "insights," occurring as a rapid flash of inspiration that connected the dots to a correct diagnosis when no symptom interpretation was obvious.

Although traditional thinking warns doctors not to trust their intuition, the researchers pointed out, "Physicians reported only 7 cases for which their intuitions turned out to be incorrect," and came to the conclusion, "There cannot be a simple, catchall directive to physicians to avoid intuition."[6]

Nurses are some of the most intuitive people I have ever met. Studies show that nurses regard their intuition highly and consider it to be a rich source of knowledge. For more than 30 years, they have contributed an abundance of literature on the use of intuition in the clinical setting.[7]

Integrative holistic nursing pioneers Barbara Dossey and Lynn Keegan make a case for intuition as an essential nursing skill.[8] In *Holistic Nursing: A Handbook for Practice*, they describe it as, "A 'gut feeling' that something is wrong or that we should do something, even if there is no real evidence to support that feeling."

An exhaustive review of 16 studies on the use of intuition in nursing examined the evidence.[9] Some of the findings included the following:

- Nurses use their intuition throughout a range of nursing duties, such as patient care, observation and documentation.
- Nurses understand that their intuitions about patients may have no obvious or logical reasons.
- Intuitive nurses report making non-verbal, non-physical "energetic contact" with patients.
- Nurses use intuition in deciding which actions to take and tasks to perform.
- The use of intuition helps increase a nurse's sense of self-confidence.

The researchers summarized, "We find that intuition plays a key role in more or less all of the steps in the nursing process as a base for decision-making that supports safe patient care, and is a validated component of nursing clinical care expertise."

Is It Really Intuition?

It is clear that the medical world values intuition. Yet science demands that there must be a reasonable and acceptable explanation. Scientists speculate that the intuitive process taps into an expert clinician's vast knowledge base gathered from their many years in practice.[10] This knowledge, stored deep in subconscious memory, can be accessed in a non-linear, non-analytic fashion, leading to a "hunch" that may steer them to the correct diagnosis. Though this seems plausible, it also implies that only experienced practitioners have access to intuition, and that novices do not.

The idea that less experienced practitioners have no access to their intuition has been challenged. Torsten Liem, Joint Principal of the German School of Osteopathy, considers it "highly likely" that intuitive judgment in clinical reasoning contributes to the final decisions of both novices and experts.[11]

A report published in the *Journal of Holistic Nursing* investigated this notion further.[12] Researchers chose nurses with varying levels of experience from several different clinical units in one medical center. The nurses completed the Rew Intuitive Judgment Scale (RIJS).[13] Regardless of their self-reported proficiency or years in the field, no differences in their intuition scores were found. Among the nurses I've taught, I have also seen that their length of time in nursing does not have an influence on their ability to learn and use medical intuition.

Pattern recognition is another way intuition has typically been explained.[14] This is defined as the right brain's capacity to pick up and respond to both subtle and complex signals. Patterns in body language, voice tone and other physical or emotional cues that may go unnoticed by the practitioner's conscious mind are registered subconsciously, which can lead to a sense of intuitive awareness.

These two comfortable definitions of intuition – as knowledge gained from expert-level experience or as subconscious recognition of subtle cues and responses – do not accurately explain the enigmatic nature of medical intuition. While they may seem similar, they lack the crucial component of a pure, unadulterated intuitive event.

Most people are familiar with the uncanny occurrence of an out-of-the-blue intuitive hit that cannot be linked to knowledge hidden in our memories or to elusive cues lurking in our subconscious minds. Investigation into this type of phenomenon generally resides in the domain of parapsychology – a field with enough "woo-woo" in it to make a medical scientist blush. Will these two areas of science ever meet in the middle? Medical intuition may be the bridge.

Breaking New Ground: Research on Medical Intuition

In healthcare, a profession where your loftiest credentials define who you are, medical intuition does not conform. Medical intuitives come from all walks of life and from all educational backgrounds. Some have clinical training and some do not. Some developed their intuition naturally and some studied with a spiritual teacher or mentor. Others feel that their intuitive abilities were passed down through their family line. (I recall my mother regaling me with stories of my grandparents, the neighborhood healers!) Still others discovered their intuitive gifts as an aftermath of a traumatic event or through supernatural-style encounters. But no matter how intuition may have been developed, testing and validating it has proved to be a challenging task.

There are thousands of anecdotal stories about medical intuition, but surprisingly few studies have ever been conducted. Most of the published research has been in the form of case reports or qualitative studies.

As I explored the literature, one consistent type of comment caught my attention. Many of the physicians and scientists who created, participated in or reviewed the experiments became intrigued by medical intuition's extraordinary potential to transform healthcare. Their foresight is validating and their optimism is encouraging.

You will see the word "diagnosis" incorrectly used in some of the following studies. As noted in Chapter 2, Dr. Daniel Benor has provided the more accurate term "intuitive assessment."[15]

Additionally, the words "psychic" and "healer" are prevalent in the older studies. I have replaced these with the terms "medical intuitive" or "intuitive."

Assessing the Accuracy of Medical Intuition

As a professional medical intuitive, I've gauged my success by the testimonials of happy clients. I was curious to know if an empirical test for medical intuition was even possible. As I delved into the available research, it became apparent that a robust evidence base was severely lacking. Study designs were wildly inconsistent and sometimes faulty, in some cases because of a basic misunderstanding of the intuitive process. Because the literature was sparse, I set out to create an exploratory study.

My teaching system is designed to be measurable and repeatable.[16] I knew it worked – my students hit their marks and clients always gave them glowing praise – but I wanted more proof.

In Chapter 2, I introduced you to my study, "Assessing the Accuracy of Medical Intuition," which took place over eight months, concluding in March 2019.[17] The 67 self-selected subjects included a cohort of patients from UCSD Health at the University of California, San Diego, and the Cardiac Treatment Center at Scripps Memorial Hospital, La Jolla, California.

Five graduates of The Practical Path Medical Intuitive Training Practitioner Certification Program took part in the study: a registered nurse; a licensed acupuncturist; a certified functional nutritional therapy practitioner; a certified integrative nutrition coach; and a certified educator. The sessions were performed privately by phone or over the internet. No health intake was conducted, so the medical intuitives were blinded to the subjects' health issues and medical histories. The practitioners' eyes were closed throughout the sessions as well, giving them an additional level of "blindness," as the subjects' body language and facial expressions could not be seen. In addition, the medical intuitives were instructed to keep their comments solely to what they perceived during the scans.

A standardized method of intuition was used to scan the subjects' physical body systems and biofields. The practitioners also viewed "scenes" from the subjects' life histories that were intuitively identified as relevant to the physical issues. After the session, the subjects completed an online, anonymous Likert-scale survey, with a range from "strongly disagree," to "strongly agree." The results included the following:

- 94 per cent agree/strongly agree the medical intuitive accurately located their main physical issue.
- 100 per cent (of 86 per cent of subjects who completed this question) agree/strongly agree the medical intuitive accurately located their secondary physical issue.
- 94 per cent agree/strongly agree the medical intuitive accurately evaluated their health issue(s).
- 98 per cent agree/strongly agree the medical intuitive accurately described their life events.
- 93 per cent agree/strongly agree the medical intuitive accurately made a clear connection between their life events and their health issues.
- 94 per cent (of 49 per cent of subjects who had a known medical diagnosis) rated the medical intuitive as consistent/totally consistent with their known diagnosis.
- 100 per cent agree/strongly agree the medical intuitive offered useful recommendations for their health issues and concerns.
- 99 per cent were satisfied/extremely satisfied with the session.
- 97 per cent would recommend medical intuition to others.
- 96 per cent would have another session, if given the opportunity.

Subjects' comments included:

- *"Professional and informative, a very positive experience."*
- *"Very interesting session. [The medical intuitive's] comments affirmed what my surgeons, MD, and physical therapist have said to me."*
- *"Spot on. Interestingly, I had just discussed some of the items [the medical intuitive] brought up earlier today with my doctor. The session validated some of the avenues I have been exploring."*
- *"An image that was brought up in the session gave me a very helpful picture of where my issues began."*
- *"Insightful, enlightening, empowering and a lot of fun to see all the levels of mind, body, and soul's influence on health."*

It was also interesting to discover how simply hearing the information had a positive effect on the subjects' mood and perspective about their health issues. We were pleased to read comments such as:

- *"After [the medical intuitive] was done I felt a great sense of relief and confidence. She made a positive impact on my life."*
- *"I found the session helpful for providing visual metaphors for emotional issues I was experiencing, and those visualizations helped me to feel less overwhelmed."*
- *"The medical intuitive was very clear with her assessments. I felt comfortable and relaxed."*
- *"The medical intuitive hit right on certain things that I did not even know were affecting me still. Once they were brought forward, things started making so much sense. I can already tell a huge difference in my body. I am so thankful, grateful and excited!"*

These results suggest that trained and qualified medical intuitives have high subjectively reported accuracy rates in locating and evaluating primary and secondary health concerns, consistency with medical diagnoses, and are able to identify the unique life events that may have led to a person's health imbalances. The findings also show that people find medical intuition both acceptable and empowering.

As previously noted, this study was published in the *Journal of Alternative and Complementary Medicine* (*JACM*), co-authored by Dr. Paul J. Mills. As of this writing, it represents the most recent research on medical intuition published in the US. These outcomes confirm the strong need for more scientific research on medical intuition with well-funded studies. Our hope is that these promising results will support that effort.

A Double-Blind Study Sheds Light

The Science of Consciousness annual conference is a bustling, heady affair. Sponsored by the University of Arizona, Tucson, scientists and consciousness enthusiasts come from all over the world to listen to some of the great academic minds debate how to quantify the intangible nature of conscious reality. At the 2006 event, a quietly revolutionary study, "Remote Diagnosis of Medical Conditions: A Double-Blind Experiment of Medical Intuition," was presented by psychologist Sheryl Attig and Gary E. Schwartz, professor, psychologist and Director of the University of Arizona's Laboratory for Advances in Consciousness and Health.[18]

A group of seven medical intuitives, who were proficient in various methods, were recruited. The subjects were 19 congestive heart failure patients, with a control group of their 19 spouses who did not have congestive heart failure. Medical details were collected from both the patients and their spouses. The medical intuitives were given only the subjects' names, dates of birth, gender and their city and state. They were then asked to give a remote diagnosis for each subject.

The results showed that the medical intuitives were able to distinguish between healthy subjects and seriously ill subjects. They were also able to list symptoms and comorbid conditions associated with congestive heart failure. Two cardiologists reviewed the intuitives' findings and were able to determine, with a high level of accuracy, which subjects had congestive heart failure and which did not.

The study concluded, "Medical intuition appears to be a real phenomenon, worthy of further research. With further validation, it could be used as an adjunct tool for diagnosing patients, especially in difficult cases."[19] The authors commented that training for physicians and other practitioners in medical intuition could prove to be of great benefit.

Intuitive Investigators

In the previous chapter, you learned about some of the notable contributions of Edgar Cayce, who documented more than 14,000 intuitive sessions while in a hypnotic trance. Of his readings, 63 per cent were conducted specifically for physical health issues. After his death in 1945, Cayce's sons randomly selected 150 cases to be analyzed. Based on positive patient responses, they rated Cayce's accuracy at 85 per cent, comparing it favorably to the success rate of modern-day physicians.[20]

In her 1967 book, *Breakthrough to Creativity*, psychiatrist Shafica Karagulla (1914–1986) presented perhaps some of the first contemporary research in the field.[21] Her investigation of intuitive phenomena, which she named "Higher Sense Perception," contributed greatly to the current understanding of meta-sensory skills. In her book, she described her work with "sensitives" who could accurately discern health issues in the physical body and biofield.

Dr. Karagulla's vision for the future of medicine included medical intuitives as part of a clinical team assisting physicians with diagnoses and treatment choices. She envisioned medical intuitive doctors being able to discuss their findings openly and without stigma. She also anticipated intuitives playing an important part in the acceleration of scientific and technological advancements. Dr. Karagulla's inspirational ideas embody the goals of the existing research, and inform the research to come.

One of the most respected advocates of medical intuition is Dr. C. Norman Shealy (*see* Chapter 3). His long-standing interest in intuitive research helped bring the field into the public's awareness. In an initial trial, he worked with 8 intuitives and 17 patients.[22] Without engaging in any dialogue or questioning, each intuitive observed a subject in person and answered a series of questions. Dr. Shealy found the intuitives to be 98 per cent accurate in evaluating the subjects' personal and psychological issues and 80 per cent accurate in assessing physical conditions.

In a second study, Dr. Shealy personally examined and diagnosed a group of patients.[23] Six intuitives were given a photo of the patients with names and birthdates only, and were then asked to determine the primary causes of illness, and the location of any physical pain. Dr. Shealy found that for the primary causes of illness, the intuitives' accuracy ranged from 30 per cent to 65 per cent. For the location of pain, two intuitives were 75 per cent accurate, and a third was 70 per cent accurate.

Dr. Shealy's most famous collaboration was with medical intuitive Caroline Myss, who went on to achieve international acclaim. Giving her only the patients' names and dates of birth, he gauged Myss's accuracy rate at 93 per cent, as compared to his own diagnoses.[24] In *The Creation of Health*, Dr. Shealy states that physicians are usually 80 per cent accurate in their diagnoses but acknowledges that determining exact diagnoses for various types of illnesses can be challenging.[25] He also points out that many diagnostic tests hold significant health risks to patients. Dr. Shealy suggests, "The opinion of two or three talented intuitives could help us avoid risky diagnostic tests and help both the physician and patient rest more comfortably in the knowledge that everything reasonable has been done to make the proper diagnosis."[26]

Intuition and the Western Medicine Paradigm

When debunkers cast a skeptical eye on medical intuition, they often point to a decades-old study, published in *JACM*.[27] While the parameters of the study failed to prove clear evidence, the article set off a few rounds of fireworks in scientific circles and generated strongly worded rebuttals from respected medical experts.

Medical anthropologist David Young and physician Steven Aung undertook an experiment with three intuitives to see if they could assess medical conditions in five of Dr. Aung's patients. Four of the patients had known serious health issues, and one healthy subject was used as the control. The intuitives read each of the patients individually, using their own methods. The patient sat behind a screen during the evaluation. At the end of the session, the screen was removed and the intuitives were given the opportunity to ask questions of each patient. The intuitives' notes were then compared to the patient's medical records, along with any new information from the closing interview.

The results were not encouraging, as the intuitives had a low combined average accuracy rate of 9.4 per cent. Though there were some correlations to the patients' health issues, the authors concluded that "psychic diagnosis" was of limited value in medicine.

So, was this study a complete failure? Not exactly. In an accompanying commentary, Donald G. Murphy, a retired NIH scientist, argued that it was unfairly framed within the biased paradigm of Western medicine.[28] He pointed out that the researchers had discounted several substantial observations made by the intuitives that would have been easy to corroborate, such as diabetes, leg pain or headaches. Dr. Murphy compared the intuitives' perceptions to how physicians might use their own intuition, referring to it as "the art of medicine."

Dr. Murphy wrote, "What emerges from this study is that a hypothetical physician-psychic team has the remarkable potential of bringing missed and undiagnosed conditions to the fore. The physician member of this team would have the final responsibility for the diagnosis and treatment." Proposing training for both parties as a key component, he supported this collaborative model as both a time-saving and cost-saving strategy.

The Young and Aung article also drew a strong critical response from *JACM*'s editor-in-chief, physician Kim A. Jobst.[29] Calling out the authors' conclusions as premature and even irresponsible, he pointed out the weaknesses and narrow focus of the study design, and questioned the criteria used to validate the procedures and the outcomes. Dr. Jobst argued that the alternative medical community has a duty to investigate intuitive phenomena rigorously. He wrote, "If psychic diagnosis can be shown to be accurate, reliable and communicable, the implications are profound."

In a Letter to the Editor response to the Young and Aung report, Larry Burk, a holistic radiologist and author, offered a noteworthy story from his own career regarding a young patient and a consultation with a medical intuitive.[30] An MRI revealed a suspected malignant tumor in the girl's left sacrum and lower spine, and a biopsy was scheduled. Dr. Burk had recently met medical intuitive Caroline Myss at a conference where she had presented her work on medical intuition.[31] He took the opportunity to call Myss for a consultation on the case.

With only the name and age of the patient, Myss correctly identified the tumor location and confirmed it as malignant. She perceived a number of causes, including family relationships, genetic factors and an imbalance in the patient's second chakra. Later, the biopsy led to a diagnosis of Ewing's sarcoma, and the patient's doctors confirmed much of the life history Myss had intuited. Dr. Burk was amazed and impressed at the speed, accuracy and depth of Myss's assessment.

Putting the Puzzle Together

Psychotherapist, author and Founding Diplomate of the American Board of Integrative Holistic Medicine, Dr. Daniel

Benor is a highly respected leader in the field of subtle energy research.

In a 1992 pilot study, he and physician Jean Galbraith tested eight energy healing practitioners who claimed they were able to discern health issues by viewing colors in the aura.[32] The intuitives observed four patients with known diagnoses and wrote down their interpretations of the colors in each patient's auric field. The findings showed more gaps than overlaps in their reviews. Dr. Benor compared this to the old adage of the blind men and the elephant – each intuitive had relayed a different piece of the "puzzle." Even so, the patients confirmed that they resonated with the vast majority of the readings.

Drs. Benor and Galbraith repeated the procedure several months later, using two patients with known diagnoses and four intuitive practitioners with excellent reputations for their aura-reading abilities.[33] This time, the intuitives were also asked to mark areas on an outline figure of the human body for perceptions of physical imbalances. The intuitives read more accurately for personal life issues, particularly early childhood traumas, than physical issues. But, just as it happened in the prior study, the patients related deeply to the intuitives' assessments.

Seeing the Patterns in Pain

Can an intuitive detect the location of spine abnorm-alities and pain simply by observing an individual's biofield? In 2002, at the Alliance Institute for Integrative Medicine in Cin-cinnati, Ohio, a small yet intriguing study aimed to find out.[34]

Researchers recruited 14 patients, all of whom had issues in a single disk of their lower spine between L1 and S1. Two healthy subjects were brought in as controls. All 16 participants were given an MRI scan. On an outline figure of the human body, they were then asked to draw where they felt their pain. Radiologists interpreted the MRI scans, noting the locations of the patients' bulging disks.

Two practitioners – one of whom was Rev. Rosalyn L. Bruyere, a respected clairvoyant and energy practitioner – were asked to evaluate the subjects' biofields. No MRI information or health history was given to the intuitives, and no communication was allowed. After a short session lasting five to ten minutes each, the medical intuitives then marked their impressions on a separate outline figure drawing.

In analyzing the results, researchers noted that the intuitives "Correctly identified disk pathology and pain patterns in a significant number of patients."[35] What they found most striking were the correlations between the pain drawings made by the medical intuitives and those made by the patients. By observing the biofield, the intuitives were able to create a precise depiction of the patients' subjective pain. The authors concluded, "The practitioners' measurements appeared to correlate both the subjective feeling of pain, a physiologic process, and an anatomical abnormality."[36]

The researchers emphasized that medical intuition could be particularly useful in detecting pain in patients who may not be able to verbally describe their symptoms. They also remarked that medical intuition could be valuable if taught and integrated into healthcare.

A Final Note on the Research

A number of other studies have been published – some with favorable outcomes and some with no significant findings. Additional information is included in the endnotes.[37]

Throughout all of the studies, regardless of the results, one powerful idea resonates: trained and qualified medical intuitives would be a profound asset in healthcare. Considering the potential benefits acknowledged in these studies, it is astounding that we do not already have years of gold-standard research to draw upon. When the medical world is ready to embrace the possibilities of medical intuition, the advantages to medicine, science and health will be endless.

CHAPTER 5

MEDICAL INTUITION IN ACTION: ESTABLISHING A NEW PARADIGM

The good physician treats the disease; the great physician treats the patient who has the disease.

Sir William Osler, Founder, Johns Hopkins Hospital

I am forever amazed by the ways in which my students apply medical intuition in their work. They are excited to be at the forefront of a new paradigm in healthcare, and many are using their skills to expand the boundaries of their fields. Traditionally, though, medical intuitives have worked at the fringes as acceptance into mainstream medicine has been slow. However, when I saw the remarkable results of a national survey, I knew a shift was in progress. If you recall, it was found that 82 per cent of medical intuitives directly assist licensed healthcare providers, 86 per cent are referred by licensed healthcare providers, and 30 per cent are licensed healthcare providers themselves.[1]

Is medical intuition to remain the best-kept secret in the medical world? Or are we ready to bring medical intuitives out of the shadows and welcome them as key members of a complete care team?

An additional question was asked of the subjects in my study (*see* Chapter 4). We wanted to know who they thought had a better understanding of their health issues and concerns: their primary healthcare provider, the medical intuitive, or both?

Their answers were eye-opening. We found that 55 per cent of the subjects chose "both;" 29 per cent felt the medical intuitive understood their issues better than their own doctors; and only 3 per cent thought their doctors understood their issues better than the medical intuitive.

Should the medical community be worried? Not at all. The answer lies in the majority of the responses. People felt that both their doctor and the medical intuitive can be equally trusted to understand them. These findings illustrate the potential for acceptable and open collaborative relationships between doctors and medical intuitives.

The Physician–Medical Intuitive Partnership

There are many examples of successful partnerships between physicians and medical intuitives. Throughout his career, Edgar Cayce worked closely with doctors.[2] Homeopath Wesley Ketchum's research with Cayce was presented to the American Society of Clinical Research in 1910. Regarding Cayce's abilities, Ketchum said, "I have used him in about 100 cases, and to date have never known of any error in diagnosis."[3]

In *The Doctor and the Psychic*, Leon Curry, a physician from Metter, Georgia, wrote about his long-term association with medical intuitive Greta Alexander. By examining ink prints of a patient's hands, Alexander could identify their health issues with extraordinary accuracy.[4]

As you have read, Dr. C. Norman Shealy and medical intuitive Caroline Myss have written extensively about their work together.[5]

Here are several more doctor–intuitive alliances.

A Trusted Intuitive

Physician and educator Leonard A. Wisneski is a Clinical Professor of Medicine at George Washington University Medical Center, and adjunct faculty at Georgetown University in Washington, DC. As Chair Emeritus of the Integrative Health

Policy Consortium (IHPC), he and his colleagues advocate for policy to ensure the future of integrative healthcare. His authoritative textbooks have helped form the basis of integrative health education throughout the world.

Dr. Wisneski wrote about his work with a medical intuitive in *The Scientific Basis of Integrative Health*.[6] (He also recounts his transformative story in the foreword of this book.) He describes how a medical doctor and medical intuitive can work together for patients who present complex and confounding symptoms.

> Dr. Wisneski diagnosed severe prostatitis for his patient. When the patient's fever and inflammation did not abate, he consulted a medical intuitive. The medical intuitive's assessment led him in an additional direction, allowing him to diagnose a rare thyroid condition that would have otherwise gone undetected. Dr. Wisneski wrote, "If it were not for [the medical intuitive's] reading, I never would have investigated for a thyroid disorder or have been able to assist ... in such a comprehensive manner. ... I have come to fully believe in her ability to make accurate observations – repeatedly."

Our field is indebted to Dr. Wisneski as a champion for awareness and acceptance of medical intuition in complementary and integrative health (CIH).

A Deeper View

An article titled "Expanding Diagnostic Vision with Medical Intuition," published in the December 2000 issue of *Alternative and Complementary Therapies*, featured an interview with Abraham C. Kuruvilla, an integrative family medicine doctor, and Jay Caliendo, a medical intuitive.[7] Although Dr. Kuruvilla was initially skeptical, their professional association began when

Caliendo intuitively read one of his patients with "100 per cent accuracy."

In the article, Caliendo described seeing the body as a series of layers, similar to X-ray images. He also saw the patient's energetic "biography" and information about where an illness may have originated. Dr. Kuruvilla then used his allopathic and integrative medicine knowledge to interpret Caliendo's reading. He noted that Caliendo routinely reached the same diagnoses as expensive and time-consuming tests.

The article included several impressive case studies. A dramatic example was the case of a 32-year-old woman with persistent abdominal pain.

Based on CT scan and ultrasound imaging, the suspected diagnosis was cancer of the bile duct, and a biopsy was recommended. Caliendo perceived that scarring from a seat-belt injury several years earlier had caused the bile duct to stricture, which was generating the pain in the woman's abdomen. Although the patient had told all of her doctors about the accident, only Caliendo pointed this out as relevant to her symptoms. An endoscopic procedure showed an obvious scar in the duct, and the biopsy was called off.

Dr. Kuruvilla stated that medicine needs more medical intuitives like Jay Caliendo.

A Close Collaboration

A groundbreaking model of a successful physician–intuitive team can be seen in the practice of physician Mary Coan and her working relationship with medical intuitive Wil Alaura.

I met Dr. Coan at the 2019 Integrative Health Symposium in New York. As it so often happens at conferences, I find myself being drawn to just the right people to meet. We struck up a conversation while waiting in line at the lunch buffet. When I told her I was a medical intuitive, her eyes lit up. Over lunch, I was thrilled to hear how she worked closely with Alaura, and how their collaboration had vitally enhanced her healthcare practice. Recently, I had the opportunity to reconnect with Dr. Coan, and learn more about her and Alaura's unique process.

Dr. Coan is an integrative family medicine physician at Clifton Springs Hospital in Clifton Springs, New York. For more than ten years, she and Alaura have developed a strong and effective partnership.

Alaura joins Dr. Coan and the patient in the examination room, either in person or by teleconference. As the patient describes their symptoms, Dr. Coan and Alaura work in tandem to bounce observations and ideas off each other. As an integrative physician, Dr. Coan has access to both conventional and holistic-based options. Together, they create a highly personalized care plan for the patient.

Alaura uses a range of medical intuitive skills, including claircognizance, clairvoyance and clairaudience (*see* Chapter 8). He assists Dr. Coan by discerning which options may be most energetically aligned for the patient, helping to fine-tune various interventions. Finally, they determine if the whole treatment package needs any additional adjustments. The process, which they describe as "seamless," takes approximately 45 minutes. After every session, Alaura provides the doctor with a written report of his assessment for each patient.

A potent example of their teamwork can be seen with Dr. Coan's Lyme disease patients. Lyme disease is both difficult to diagnose and to treat, as it often presents with co-infections. What may work for one patient may not work for another. The typical medical model of trying various medications over a period of weeks or months is time-consuming and expensive, and it can take a toll on a patient's health and wellbeing. In working with Alaura, Dr. Coan is able to efficiently determine which treatments will be most effective from the start. They both believe this system has brought remarkable success for patients.

Dr. Coan admits that support from her colleagues for her unorthodox methods has not been very forthcoming. In our first meeting, I asked what keeps her going in the face of skepticism. "It's simple," she said. "My patients get better."

She believes the growing interest in energy-based methods is driven by people for whom mainstream healthcare has failed. Dr. Coan describes her work with Alaura as the bridge between conventional and holistic medicine. "Patients have a lot of interest in working with a provider who is open to more holistic options. They may have been looking for help for years and getting nowhere. Now they have a whole new way of experiencing healthcare. We give them hope," she says. Alaura adds, "We give them results."

Dr. Coan's patients emphatically agree. I was able to interview several of them for this book. Each talked about how they felt included in their healthcare process and how the doctor–medical intuitive relationship inspired confidence in this unconventional model. Here are three notable cases:

Amy suffered from recurrent bouts of thyroid cancer, which required annual surgeries. Her doctors had no explanation for why the cancer persisted and offered no other treatment options. "It felt like my doctors were just throwing a dart and hoping for the best. I would have done anything to heal, and standard medicine wasn't helping," Amy said. Dr. Coan and Alaura created a treatment plan using a range of protocols. In the seven years since she began working with them, Amy has not had an issue with her thyroid. "I can't imagine approaching my health any other way," she said.

Claire was dealing with a myriad of debilitating health challenges, as well as painful emotions due to heavy personal losses. In her first meeting with Dr. Coan and Alaura, she was impressed by their combination of medical training and energetic information. Claire felt a growing sense of confidence in the way they looked at her issues from both the physical and emotional perspectives. "They were interested in knowing me holistically. They offered options and points of view that you wouldn't get from a standard medical doctor," she said. "Dr. Coan and Wil are respectful of each other's practice, which is a huge benefit for me as a patient because I receive the value of what they both bring to the table. It's so comprehensive."

"They saved my life," Bethany said. Bedridden and paralyzed, Bethany had received a correct diagnosis of Lyme disease by a specialist and had been put on a long-term series of antibiotics. Unfortunately, none of the medications were working and, worse, severe chemical sensitivities made it difficult for her to tolerate them. "I was afraid that if I went off the antibiotics I would end up bedridden again," she said. "I couldn't keep taking them, but I couldn't stay on them anymore. It was a terrifying situation." Dr. Coan and Alaura worked together to find the right combination of antibiotics, supplements and dosages that would work for her. Had it not been for this unique alliance, Bethany feels she would not have survived.

Clinician as Medical Intuitive

If you are a practitioner, you may be wondering how medical intuition could be integrated into your own practice. Perhaps you are questioning your ability to use intuitive skills yourself. Here are perspectives from a medical doctor and a critical care nurse, both of whom are also medical intuitives.

The Intuitive Physician

Though medical intuition was not a new concept to family medicine physician Lloyd Costello, he was convinced that one had to be born with the ability and that it certainly could not be learned. When he heard me speak at a holistic health event, he was immediately drawn to the idea when I told the audience, "Anyone can learn how to develop their intuition." The next day, he enrolled in my program.

Dr. Costello feels strongly that medical intuition can help open up new avenues for preventive care. "Being a physician who is also a medical intuitive, I can intervene before symptoms manifest and work toward a preventive treatment," he said. He points out that patients often forget to tell their doctor about a symptom, or focus on a particular health concern, when other, perhaps more critical, issues may be present. Also, a patient may believe a problem they have learned to live with is perfectly normal, when it may be an early symptom of something more serious. "In wellness visits, I can intuitively screen for any potential conditions that may not have reached the symptomatic stage. For example, a symptom, such as constipation, may not be seen as abnormal to the patient. With medical intuition, I can pinpoint these kinds of hidden or unspoken issues in the examination process," he stated.

Dr. Costello is particularly interested in helping address emotional and lifestyle considerations that may be affecting a patient's health. "'Lower your stress for hypertension,' is a typical thing a doctor might say. That's very vague," he pointed out.

The medical intuitive doctor, however, would be able to intuitively perceive where the stress is coming from – work, family life or other stressors. From here the doctor can assess how that stress is affecting the patient. "Are they losing sleep? Are they not eating well? Or are they not taking steps to calm their mind and body? This type of information would be beneficial to know if the patient needs to see a specialist, such as a counselor, psychotherapist, psychiatrist or coach," Dr. Costello explained.

As the public demands more alternatives, Dr. Costello sees a time when physicians using medical intuition would seldom have to say: *There is nothing more we can do for you.* "In my practice, I have never *not* seen a place for some aspect of relief for a patient, whether physical, emotional, or spiritual," Dr. Costello said. "Hopelessness only leads to depression and death. We look for the paths of healing and hope."

The Intuitive Nurse

Elizabeth Thorson, a nurse and medical intuitive consultant, worked in critical care for more than 20 years. Having been at the epicenter of life-and-death circumstances in the highly charged environments of the Emergency Room, Intensive Care Unit (ICU) and operating room, she is no stranger to the minute-by-minute drama of the unfolding stories around her. We spoke about how medical intuition has supported her nursing career.

"I would just know things in advance about a patient. When there is resuscitation going on, or when an emergency is being called, having that intuitive information would help me to discern which choices might be best for the patient, and even suggest specific tests that may not have been considered," Thorson said. "In critical care you learn to have a voice, partly because it's such a team effort." With her intuition, she was not afraid to speak up.

Thorson found that she was also able to perceive a psychological, emotional or even a spiritual emergency. "For example, I might treat a woman with bumps and bruises who said she tripped and fell. But, intuitively, I may have seen that she was shoved." This kind of information could give Thorson and the other providers the opportunity to address the bigger issue of suspected cases of domestic abuse. When she worked in the ICU, Thorson found she was able to intuit the profound spiritual decisions people made in the moments between living and dying.

These powerful experiences solidified her reputation for intuitive savvy among her colleagues. "It was not uncommon for them to ask me what I thought was really going on with a patient," she said. Thorson considers herself incredibly fortunate to have worked with an open-minded and supportive group of medical professionals.

Medical Intuition in Higher Education

In 1980, an unusual question was posed to the deans of medical schools, residents, professors and other medical faculty: "Should psychic studies be included in psychiatric education?"[8]

- 58 per cent of respondents believed that an understanding of psychic phenomena is important in psychiatric education.
- 44 per cent felt that "psychic factors" were important in the healing process.

This study, along with a more recent study from 2009, concluded that not only is there much value in including intuitive development in psychiatric education, but also that "intuition should be used to suggest, guide and modify psychiatric diagnosis."[9]

Unfortunately, intuitive development is not a subject regularly taught in medical schools. Most academic institutions would consider it an outlandish idea. However, thanks to visionary leadership in integrative, functional and holistic-based education, I have been privileged to present lectures and seminars on medical intuition to medical students, physicians, nurses and practitioners of every kind. I'm constantly delighted with the level of enthusiasm for this vital and empowering skill. A new generation of healthcare professionals agrees that medical intuition should be an essential part of health and wellness training.

It may take a while to incorporate medical intuition into the halls of higher learning. But here is a little-known account of an accomplished and courageous medical intuitive who infiltrated a university medical school's curriculum.

The Ivy League Intuitive

Winter Robinson's storied career as a medical intuitive and educator began in the early 1980s. Starting out as a forensic psychologist and analyst for the Virginia State Attorney General, her interest in all things metaphysical led her to the Monroe Institute, a center for the exploration of human consciousness, based in Faber, Virginia. She later became a staff trainer and more recently hosted her own programs there.

In the mid-1980s, Robinson was asked to teach a class for medical students at Brown University School of Medicine in Providence, Rhode Island, as part of their Physical Assessment curriculum. Two forward-thinking professors and a dean at Brown championed her classes, which she developed to train medical students, faculty and residents to perform a medical intuitive assessment. The classes were held nearby at Roger Williams Medical Center.

Students received only a patient's name and hospital room number. They were asked to write up a case report based solely on their remote intuitive assessment. Encouraged to keep their minds open, they were allowed to use their intuition in any way they chose. Afterwards, each student visited their patient and conducted an interview regarding what was intuitively "picked up" in their blind assessment. The classes were a big hit. The series began with about five students, and by the time it ended a few years later, nearly 40 students attended every class.

I spoke with psychiatric physician Frank J. Faltus, who had heard about Robinson's classes and dropped in to take part. He recalled an unforgettable experience.

Dr. Faltus was given the name of a patient who was located several floors away in the hospital. He was asked to perform an intuitive body scan using any of his senses. Dr. Faltus found himself using his mind's eye to scan through his own body. Three sensations stood out – he felt tingling in his fingers and toes, he intuitively saw an ulcer in the stomach, and he noticed a sense of confusion in the front part of his brain. Somehow, he knew the confusion was chemical in nature and not from a stroke or tumor. After his assessment, he learned that the patient had crippling arthritis of the hands and feet, which had been treated with steroids, causing both a stomach ulcer and steroid-induced psychosis.

Dr. Faltus was amazed to discover that his intuitive perceptions related directly to the patient's conditions – a regular occurrence for students in Robinson's classes. Unfortunately, none of the students' case documentation was kept or published.

While her classes ran only for a short time at Brown University, they stand as an exceptional example of what is possible in bringing the art of intuition into medical education.

Making a Case for Case Studies

Case studies are important touchstones for real-world applications of innovative methods. The following case studies demonstrate some of the unique benefits of medical intuition.

CASE STUDY: SEEING NEW SCIENCE

Medical intuitives are known for their ability to be ahead of the curve on health information that may not yet be in the public eye. It's also not unusual for a medical intuitive to identify new science that may still be in the research stage. Here is an example from my practice.

Dave sustained a hernia as a result of an emergency operation to remove a colon tumor. His hospital stay included a few weeks in the ICU, and the hernia developed several months after returning home. Dave's surgeon told him there was not an immediate need, but recommended that he consider another surgery using surgical mesh to fix the hernia. Dave was concerned about possible complications of hernia mesh and called me in October 2018 for a consultation.

During our session, I intuitively perceived that a recent experimental study on hernia mesh had taken place in a foreign country, and had reported positive results. The research investigated a process of coating the mesh with a patient's own stem cells to help the body accept it more easily, lowering the risk of post-surgery rejection and inflammation. Neither Dave nor I had ever heard of this procedure, and his surgeon had not mentioned it.

After the session, I searched online for any information about what I had just intuited. I found a study from a Chinese university on the successful use of hernia mesh in rats.[10] Published in September 2018, just one month prior to our session, the report detailed the use of adipose-derived stem cells to coat hernia mesh, reducing rejection and inflammation. I contacted Dave with this information and encouraged him to bring it to his doctor's attention.

CASE STUDY: BALL AND SOCKET

Stephanie Valenzuela is a licensed allied health provider and a certified graduate of my program. In this case study, she fielded a common client question and assisted with an excellent outcome.

The pain in Valerie's hip was getting worse. After meeting with her doctor, Valerie was faced with the decision of whether or not to have hip replacement surgery. She decided to have a session with Stephanie to see if a medical intuitive assessment could provide some helpful information. Stephanie explained that she was not able to advise Valerie on medical decisions and that she should consult with her doctor.

Stephanie then intuitively scanned Valerie's right hip. She immediately saw the word *impingement* over the area and discerned that the hip joint did not form correctly during Valerie's childhood development. She observed the ball of the joint slipping out of alignment in the socket, as it didn't appear to hold in place. She also perceived that Valerie's doctor would be able to see the full nature of the misalignment during a surgery if Valerie chose to have it.

Valerie decided to move ahead with the procedure. Afterwards, she excitedly told Stephanie that the doctor had confirmed everything Stephanie had intuited. There was an impingement in the hip, as the ball and socket had not formed correctly in childhood. She even sent Stephanie a photo of the hip joint that was removed. Valerie credits the medical intuitive session as giving her clear insight into her health issue and appreciated the opportunity to hear her body's messages.

CASE STUDY: A DENTIST'S DISTRESS

Biologist, author and educator Cay Randall-May is a respected medical intuitive with an illustrious career of more than 30 years. She uses her skills in client consultations and in rigorous research in biofield science.[11] Dr. Randall-May shared a memorable case of a dentist with a mysterious heart problem.

Dr. Randall-May gave her client, Dr. Anderson, a telephone reading in July 1999. Despite having a healthy and active lifestyle, he had undergone five coronary bypass surgeries. His doctors had chalked his cardiac issues up to "stress."

"In our session, I intuitively saw that he had an infection with a *Chlamydia bacterium*, probably *pneumoniae*. I also detected that he might have caught the infection by inhaling aerosolized bacteria in the course of treating his dental patients," Dr. Randall-May recalled. At the time Dr. Anderson acquired the infection, dentists did not generally wear protective masks, and airborne infections were considered an occupational hazard.

Her client relayed this information to his physician, who was skeptical but agreed to do the appropriate tests. To his physician's surprise, the tests returned positive and Dr. Anderson was placed on a course of antibiotics. "My client's physician asked what prompted him to request such a test, and he told the doctor about our intuitive consultation," Dr. Randall-May said. "It is now 2021, and Dr. Anderson has not had a recurrence of arterial blockage."

CASE STUDY: A SIMPLER SOLUTION FOR SINUSES

Holly Scalmanini is an acupuncturist and medical intuitive. While treating a patient's stubborn cough, she noticed that her usual remedies were not working. Holly offered her patient a medical intuitive session, which pinpointed the source of the problem.

Jill came to see Holly with a persistent cough she'd been suffering with for eight months. Some months before, Jill had dealt with a bout of bronchitis and a sinus infection, which were treated with antibiotics. Holly's acupuncture treatments and herbs helped, but the cough still persisted.

When Holly looked at Jill's health with medical intuition, she determined that the cough was secondary to issues with Jill's sinuses and respiratory system, which were unable to function properly due to a variety of environmental allergens in her home.

"I could intuitively see mold and mildew in her basement and old, dusty carpeting on the stairs leading to the main floor, both of which were exacerbating her cough," Holly said. She also discerned that Jill's symptoms would be relieved by moving her home office out of the basement and upstairs into the main living area.

After the session, samples were taken from the basement and carpet for testing. The results confirmed a mold infestation in the basement and allergens in the carpeting. Jill moved her office upstairs and her cough went away."

JOURNAL EXERCISE FOR PRACTITIONERS

Can you relate any of the case studies to a recent client or patient visit from your wellness practice? Where might medical intuition have been a valuable skill in understanding their health issue? How might medical intuition help you intuitively discern more ways to assist your client or patient?

CHAPTER 6

THE MIND–BODY CONNECTION

The spirit is the master, imagination the tool, and the body the plastic material.

Paracelsus

My Healing Story

"The biopsy is negative but I'd like to remove the tumor anyway, just in case," my doctor said. It was dysplasia, a non-cancerous growth. "We can schedule the surgery for two weeks ahead." I agreed, feeling very relieved.

"Doctor, would you mind if I practiced meditating to see if I can make it go away?" I asked, fully expecting her to laugh me out of her office. "I just read a book by Dr. Deepak Chopra, and I want to see if his suggestions will work for me."

The doctor tilted her head and looked at me as if I had just said I had irrefutable proof that the moon was made of green cheese. "What book is that?" she asked. "Quantum Healing," I replied. "He shows people how to use their minds to heal their bodies." With a bemused smile, she said she didn't think it would hurt me and sent me on my way

For the next two weeks, every morning after my meditation practice, I did a short visualization technique I'd read about in Dr. Chopra's book. I wanted to find an image that would make me smile while I imagined the unwanted growth dissolving away. Instinctively, I knew that my body would respond better to a positive image than to a negative one. I wasn't worried – in fact, I didn't feel any emotion about the tumor at all, other than a curiosity to experiment with this new idea and see what might happen.

I imagined happy, giggling soap bubbles and a cheerful scrub brush, joyfully cleaning up the area and leaving my body sparkling clean. It was easy to do, and it was fun! I told myself to not worry about the outcome.

Two weeks later, as I was shivering slightly in the thin hospital gown, the doctor came in to examine me. I heard her gasp. "What is it?" I cried, alarmed – thinking I must have done something terrible to myself. She looked at me with the same quizzical head tilt. "The tumor is half the size it was two weeks ago. What did you do?"

I'm certain you've had patients or clients with healing stories like this. You may even have had one yourself. In fact, there are many stories of "miraculous" healings far more significant than mine. But are actual miracles occurring, or do we really have the power to shift our body's physiology simply by using our thoughts?

Medical science calls these events "spontaneous remissions" or "spontaneous regressions," meaning "a reduction or disappearance of symptoms without any therapeutic intervention."[1] The term "idiopathic" means a condition that has no known medical cause. Neither of these explanations are satisfying and both ignore the undeniable link between the mind and the body.

How should the world of healthcare perceive these extraordinary events? Should they be chalked up to unexplained mysteries? Or can we learn from them? I believe that we can and we should. As we understand more about how the mind and body are connected, there is increasing scientific validation for how our minds can affect our health.

Mind–body therapies are on the rise, and science is keeping pace. A simple search on the term "mind–body medicine" in the National Institutes of Health's database yields more than 50,000 peer-reviewed studies and papers. Yoga and meditation are practiced by millions of adults and children in the US.[2] Integrative health practitioners consider mind–body methods, such as mindfulness and biofeedback, to be essential components of whole-person care.[3] Uncle Sam also approves. Breath work, guided imagery, Tai Chi and more are included in a wellness plan for US veterans.[4] There are even mind–body smartphone apps for those on the go.[5]

Definitions of "mind–body medicine" include:

- *An approach to medicine that recognizes the effect of thought, feeling and belief on health, as well as the impact of health and illness on attitude and thought.*[6]
- *Taking into account the physiological, psychic and spiritual connections between the state of the body and that of the mind.*[7]

Medical intuition perfectly aligns with these definitions. Medical intuitives can observe the innate bond between the mind and the body. And we encourage our clients to develop this bond for themselves (*see* the exercise at the end of this chapter and more in Chapter 9).

Pioneers of Mind–Body Medicine

There is much we can learn from those who have been at the forefront of mind–body medicine. These pioneers have struggled to share their knowledge within a reductionist medical paradigm. Although there are many respected authorities in the field, I am highlighting three influencers who helped shape what we know today as mind–body medicine.

Giving Cancer Patients Hope and Healing

O. Carl Simonton (1942–2009), a specialist in radiation oncology, is recognized as a game-changing innovator in the use of mind–body interventions for cancer support. He described his research into the connections between a patient's attitudes, beliefs and their state of health in his groundbreaking 1978 book, *Getting Well Again.*[8]

Dr. Simonton noticed that patients with a positive outlook had fewer side effects from their cancer treatments. He also observed that a patient's feelings of hopelessness contributed to ill health and even death.

Dr. Simonton's unconventional treatment plan for his patients included meditation, visualization and lifestyle counseling, alongside regular medical care. He found that their survival time doubled and their quality of life greatly improved. "Most of us kill ourselves with unconscious emotional pain," Dr. Simonton said. Regarding those who say there is no hope, he stated, "Label those people as ill-informed and hazardous to your health."[9]

As is the case with many of history's visionaries, Dr. Simonton's work was extremely controversial. He was ridiculed and even castigated by the medical establishment at the time. It wasn't until many years later that his dedicated research was acknowledged for its importance.[10]

One result of Dr. Simonton's contributions can be seen in the popularity of Mindfulness-Based Stress Reduction (MBSR), a therapeutic meditation technique developed by Jon Kabat-Zinn, and used as treatment support for a wide variety of chronic conditions and illnesses.[11]

Dr. Simonton's influence can also be seen in the development of lifestyle medicine – a preventive approach that emphasizes the importance of nutrition, exercise, stress reduction and healthy behaviors.[12] In a stunning confirmation in 2012, the American Medical Association urged physicians to "offer evidence-based lifestyle interventions as the first and primary mode of preventing and, when appropriate, treating chronic disease within clinical medicine."[13] I'm sure Dr. Simonton would have been proud.

A Physician of Higher Consciousness

An acclaimed expert in mind–body medicine, physician Deepak Chopra has written more than 90 books and was named by *TIME* magazine as one of the 100 icons of the 20th century.[14] Dr. Chopra is best known for his concepts of quantum healing, which he defines as "the ability of one mode of consciousness (the mind) to spontaneously correct the mistakes in another mode of consciousness (the body)."[15] He suggests that we all have the ability to change our health and longevity by deliberately accessing profound states of quantum consciousness.

Dr. Chopra points out that science is now beginning to recognize that the body is actually a "field of energy and intelligence that is inextricably connected to the mind."[16] In discussing the potentials of self-healing with his patients, he said, "You can believe the diagnosis, but not the prognosis."[17] Dr. Chopra continues to lead the field in the exploration of science and spirituality.

A Woman of Affirmation and Healing

Before Louise Hay (1926–2017) created her publishing empire, Hay House, she wrote about healing herself of cancer using meditation, forgiveness exercises and lifestyle changes. Considered a founder of the modern-day self-help movement, Hay's first two bestselling books, *Heal Your Body* and *You Can Heal Your Life*, introduced her philosophy of personal growth, self-healing and positive affirmations to the world.[18]

In the mid-1980s, Hay became a galvanizing figure in the Los Angeles AIDS community, which embraced her uplifting principles of self-care. Her life's work with Hay House has influenced generations with a worldwide platform of leading-edge experts in mind–body medicine. Hay is famously quoted as saying, "I do not fix my problems. I fix my thinking. Then the problems fix themselves."[19]

These three leading lights paved the way for a major shift in the public's awareness of mind–body health. Because their ideas are so familiar to us now, we may not realize that society had very little context for their discoveries when their work was first presented. Despite that, their contributions have changed the course of history by bringing important innovations to healthcare.

Is Medical Intuition a Placebo?

Since medical intuition is not a health treatment or intervention, it doesn't belong under the heading of a placebo. However, investigations into the placebo effect clearly demonstrate the crucial link between our thoughts and beliefs, and our potentials for healing.

The word "placebo" means "to please." Placebos look like real drugs but are made of harmless substances, such as a sugar pill or saline. In double-blind clinical trials, placebos are used to test the effectiveness of pharmaceutical drugs and treatments. In the US, all new drugs must perform better than the placebo in order to be put on the market.[20]

Obviously, taking a placebo should have no impact on the body. But the "placebo effect" happens when a placebo has a more beneficial result than the drug being tested – simply because a patient *believes* it will work.

A 2005 meta-analysis on the use of placebos for patients with irritable bowel syndrome showed effectiveness rates ranging between 16 per cent and 71.4 per cent.[21] More recent studies place placebo cure rates as high as 79 per cent.[22]

What is truly fascinating about placebos is that studies have shown:

- longer placebo treatment times and more doctor visits were more effective
- two pills gave more relief than one pill
- bigger capsules worked better than smaller capsules
- stronger discomfort or pain produced a more powerful placebo healing result.[23]

Even the color of a placebo is important – red, yellow and orange pills can create a stimulant effect, while blue and green pills are shown to be more tranquilizing.[24]

But can we really *believe* our way into feeling better? Researchers at Harvard University have found that the placebo effect is created by the relationship between the brain chemistry, the mind and the body.[25] "Happy" hormones that make us feel good, such as endorphins and dopamine, are shown to increase with the use of placebos. Perhaps the ultimate surprise is that the very same chemical reactions occur in the brain even when the patient knows they are taking a placebo![26]

Ted Kaptchuk, Professor of Medicine at Harvard Medical School and Director of the placebo studies program at Beth Israel Deaconess Medical Center in Boston, Massachusetts, explains: "The placebo effect is more than positive thinking – believing a treatment or procedure will work. It's about creating a stronger connection between the brain and body and how they work together."[27] Though controversial, some doctors are prescribing placebos for their patients for a variety of health issues.[28]

The word "nocebo" means "to harm." If our minds can create a positive outcome with a placebo, the flipside is the "nocebo effect" – an expectation of a negative outcome. In other words, if a patient is told that a procedure, drug or surgery may have harmful side effects or possible adverse results, they may begin to exhibit those very same negative symptoms. John Kelley, Deputy Director of Harvard's placebo program, notes, "Just imagining something is happening is enough to activate those portions of the brain associated with that thought, worry or pain."[29]

Over 300,000 placebo trials have been conducted worldwide on drugs, surgical procedures, medical devices and complementary therapies.[30] This exciting research is revealing exactly how our mindset can affect the specific neural mechanisms of the brain that motivate the placebo response. Studying these connections helps us to understand the mighty mind–body power of the placebo effect.

The Power of Visualization

In *Top Brain, Bottom Brain*, neuroscientist Stephen Kosslyn wrote, "Visualization activates the same neural networks that actual task performance does, which can strengthen the connection between brain and body."[31] Athletes often use mental imagery before a game to help them excel.[32] Studies have found that visualization skills can boost musicians' performance and confidence.[33] As a student in music school, I remember one of my professors encouraging us to play our scales "in our minds." I was thrilled to find that mental imagery was an excellent shortcut, and I definitely didn't miss the long hours of manual practice with the metronome.

Guided imagery and other mind–body techniques are being used to improve nearly every aspect of life, for health, business, relationships and overall happiness.[34] Research continues to confirm the efficacy of these helpful, non-invasive wellness options. Ultimately, the science points to an understanding that there is no real separation between our thoughts, our emotions and our health.

Creating an Intuitive Connection with Our Body

Our bodies have a strong desire to tell us what they want and need. By intentionally and intuitively tuning in, we can help to gently open new avenues of communication and understanding.

While you practice the following exercise, begin to notice any intuitive messages. These may show up as physical sensations, mental images, feelings, or a sense of *knowing*. You may find words or phrases popping into your mind. If you find yourself zoning out, falling asleep, feeling fidgety or distracted, please pause and take a slow, deep breath in and out. Then, gently bring your attention back to the process. Make a mental note of where in your body you were focusing when a distracting reaction occurred.

If you feel any physical or emotional discomfort during this exercise, please stop immediately and take a few deep, relaxing breaths. We want to connect with our bodies in a calm, loving and supportive way, so make sure to honor the messages your body may give you.

Give yourself time as you go through the steps. You can read the script to yourself and practice as you go. You can also have a friend read it aloud to you.

EXERCISE: SAY HELLO
TO YOUR BODY

Begin by sitting in a comfortable chair with your feet flat on the floor. Take a slow, deep breath in … and exhale.

Take another deep breath and feel the air expanding your lungs and upper chest as you breathe in. Exhale, and feel the air rushing out of your mouth or nose as you breathe out.

Now, breathe normally.

Put your attention on the soles of your feet. Say "hello!" to the soles of your feet. Notice any sensations. Do they feel warm or cool, calm or tense?

Now, put your awareness on the toes on each foot and say "hello!" to your toes. If you like, you may wiggle your toes and notice how they feel.

Next, put your attention on both feet up to your ankles. Say "hello!" to your feet. How do they feel? Just notice any sensations or intuitions.

Put your awareness on the shins and calves of your legs. Notice any physical sensations or intuitions that may come up. Say "hello!" to your calves and your shins.

Now, put your attention on your knees. Notice any sensations or intuitions in your knees. Say "hello!" to your knees.

Put your awareness on your thighs, your hips and behind. Notice how they feel against the seat and back of the chair. Say "hello!" and notice any sensations or intuitions associated with your thighs, your hips and behind.

Take a moment to thank your hips, thighs, legs and feet for doing the best job they can for you, in every moment of every day.

Now, say "hello!" to your reproductive and urinary area. Notice any intuitions or sensations.

Please put your attention on your torso up to your belly button. Say "hello!" to your intestines, your lower back and spine. Notice anything that may intuitively come up for you in these areas.

Now, put your awareness on your mid-torso. Say "hello!" to your pancreas, your spleen, your kidneys, stomach, gallbladder and liver, as well as your mid-back and spine. Pay attention to any sensations or intuitions that may come up. Thank your wonderful organs for doing the best job they can for you, in every moment of every day.

Notice if you feel sleepy, fidgety, bored or if your attention wanders. If so, take a relaxing breath in and out, and bring your attention back to your body.

Now, put your attention on your lungs, heart, chest, upper back and shoulders. Say "hello!" to this part of your body. Notice any sensations or intuitions in this area.

Please put your awareness on your fingers, palms and wrists. If you like, you may wiggle your fingers. Put your awareness on your forearms, elbows and upper arms. Say "hello!" to your arms and hands. Notice any intuitions or sensations.

Please thank your arms and hands for helping you to embrace others, lift, touch and hold, and for doing their job as best they can, in every moment.

Now, put your awareness on your neck, your jaw, tongue, teeth and mouth. Say "hello!" and notice sensations or intuitions in these areas.

Put your attention on your ears, your eyes, your nose and sinuses. Say "hello!" and give yourself a moment to notice anything present for you in these areas.

Put your awareness on your brain and say "hello!" to your brain. Thank your entire head for doing the best job it can in every moment, with sight, sound, hearing and taste.

Now, thank your whole body for doing the best job it can in every moment of every day. Thank every cell in your body for helping to keep you moving forward toward health and wellbeing.

Take one more deep breath in ... and exhale.

Journal Practice: Take a moment to write down any intuitions or sensations that came up for you in this exercise. Also make a note of any body areas where your attention might have wandered or where you may have felt sleepy or zoned out. Journaling can help you become more aware and connect more deeply to those parts of your body that may want more of your attention.

CHAPTER 7

THE ENERGETICS
OF TRAUMA

Awareness is the first step in healing.

Dean Ornish, MD

There are many types of trauma. Defined as experiences that are deeply distressing or disturbing, emotional shocks or physical injury, the word itself means "wound." Trauma can be "acute," resulting from an isolated stressful or overwhelming occurrence, such as an accident, natural disaster or a violent incident.[1] Trauma can also be "chronic," from repeated exposures to situations such as domestic violence or child abuse. "Complex" trauma can be caused by a prolonged series of traumatizing events.

Then there is "vicarious" trauma that develops from empathic connections with people who have gone through trauma themselves. Trauma can even be passed down transgenerationally, including through historical events such as war or genocide, which may create psychological and physical health effects that can span generations.[2] Post-traumatic stress disorder (PTSD), a well-studied result of trauma, can cause states of dissociation, anxiety, depression, self-destructive behaviors and more.[3]

Physicians and mental healthcare professionals work directly with a patient's physical and psychological traumas. But there is another kind of imbalance that may be hidden and linger long after the original trauma has passed – one that medical intuition is uniquely designed to assess: the *energetic damage* generated by a traumatic life event.

Energetic damage is a disturbance in the natural flow of energy within the body and biofield that can result from traumatic life events experienced in childhood, teenage or adult years, passed down through family DNA, or even stored in "past lives." Medical intuitives have described this disturbance in many ways – as an energetic signature, emotional "congestion," or a type of soul wounding.[4] Energetic damage may be observed as patterns of imbalanced, disrupted or blocked energy. These patterns can include limiting beliefs, thoughts or emotions that may be conscious or subconscious. When energetic damage reaches a tipping point, illness may manifest.

It is important to make clear that assessing energetic damage from the perspective of medical intuition is not to be considered the practice of medicine, psychotherapy, psychological advice, counseling, hypnotherapy or any alternative healing arts practice.

A basic tenet of medical intuition is that every imbalance, whether physical, emotional, mental or spiritual, has, at its root, an element of energetic damage. In his seminal book, *The Body Keeps the Score: Brain, Mind, and Body in the Healing of Trauma*, psychiatrist Bessel van der Kolk writes, "We have learned that trauma is not just an event that took place sometime in the past; it is also the imprint left by that experience on mind, brain, and body."[5] Could the "imprint" Dr. van der Kolk refers to relate to the energetic damage a medical intuitive might perceive?

Solving the Mystery of Hidden Energetic Damage

All forms of trauma can be both memorable and deeply significant. Energetic damage, however, may be far more subtle. People may even consider it inconsequential. But the impact of hidden energetic damage can often be found at the root of puzzling or persistent health or life issues.

For example, if a toddler accidentally breaks a favorite toy and gets scolded by her mother, the interaction may not create a lasting memory in the child's mind. Most people would agree that toddlers often break things, and mothers often scold. However, in a medical intuitive session with the grown woman who was once the errant toddler, this seemingly insignificant early life incident may reveal energetic damage driving a current health concern. Long-term patterns of energetic damage may also influence the way she perceives herself, others in her life, or understands "how the world works."

For most people, the critical link between our life history and our health is shrouded in mystery. For a medical intuitive, however, observing the connections between the two can be clear and obvious. The following case study is an example of a client whose hidden energetic damage in childhood created real-time consequences.

CASE STUDY: ROBERT

Robert, a successful architect in his early forties, was suffering from painful gut issues and acid reflux. His symptoms had started two years prior with multiple digestive problems, unexplained weight loss and curious rashes that would come and go.

He had lost count of the number of doctors he had consulted and tests he had taken, all of which were inconclusive, regardless of his debilitating symptoms. Robert felt conventional medicine had given up on him and that the solutions his doctors had provided – primarily pharmaceutical options – were not solving his problems. Robert was also deeply worried about his future, as his health was impacting his enjoyment of life.

As I began intuitively viewing his physical body, I saw that his digestive system was dealing with a multi-layered gut imbalance, affecting his ability to digest and absorb nutrients from food. His lymphatic system looked like it was working very hard to maintain immune balance, and it appeared fatigued and depleted. I also saw that Robert's limbic and nervous systems were bearing much of the brunt of this stressful situation.

In asking his body what could potentially assist in healing, its first suggestion was to work with a skilled naturopathic doctor for supplements to address the reflux. His body requested well-cooked foods as a way to boost absorption, and suggested working with a nutritionist. To calm the limbic system and vagus nerve, meditation and breath-work techniques were recommended.

Robert's health issues had surfaced during a time of intense stress over the loss of an important personal project, and coincided with the death of his beloved mother. His energy showed me that he was holding emotional pain and stoicism in his gut area and in his third chakra, located in the solar plexus. I saw potential benefit from working with a grief counselor in a therapeutic setting. This was not only to grieve the painful loss of his mother, but also to allow himself to process the sadness and frustration over the changes in his own physical vitality.

When I observed where the energetic damage began, the first image I saw was of Robert at nine years old. He was attending an outdoor event at his grade school and standing in line for a bus to take the children on a field trip. There was energy and activity all around him, with the noise of kids laughing and calling. Robert, however, was feeling chilled, shaky and sick to his stomach. He wanted to cry, run to the bathroom or ask an adult for help. But he was fearful of being left behind, and deeply embarrassed to bring any unwanted attention to himself. At that instant, Robert resolved he would have to "man up" and not show any sign of weakness. He made a decision to be stoic, no matter what. Robert's decision at age nine, which was made in a powerful moment of physical and emotional distress, had embedded the energetic damage of that incident into both his third chakra and his digestive system.

The next image I saw was of Robert at age three. His mother had fallen ill with influenza and had to be quarantined for a few weeks. For the first time in Robert's young life, his mother was unavailable to him, and he was inconsolable. The loss of his mother's presence at this tender age made a deep impression and set up a chronic state of high alert in his energetic systems.

Robert and his mother were extremely close. When his mother died, she was living in another country far away from him. At her passing, his grief activated the pain of loss he faced at age three. In addition, his nine-year-old decision to bottle up his emotions contributed to the stress, setting off the imbalance in his gut.

Though Robert had no conscious memory of these two impactful scenes from his early years, this assessment showed that the energetic damage remained. He corroborated that throughout his life, whenever he felt a loss, or a fear of loss, he experienced both gut troubles and a strong drive to be stoic. Ultimately, Robert's body was asking him to become a partner in his grieving and healing process.

When Robert and I connected again, he acknowledged our session as the starting point from which he'd been able to address his health from a multifaceted perspective. He told me he had been exploring a range of mind–body and lifestyle approaches, such as acupuncture, integrative medicine, yoga and meditation, all of which he felt supported his continued wellbeing.

The Science of Trauma: Adverse Childhood Experiences, Psychoneuroimmunology and Epigenetics

Psychologists have studied the mind–body connection and the effects of childhood trauma in depth. Known as Adverse Childhood Experiences (ACEs), they include verbal, physical or sexual abuse, domestic violence, and exposure to drug or alcohol abuse.[6] Extensive research into ACEs shows direct correlations between early life trauma and later life health consequences, including cancer, heart disease, respiratory illness, mental health issues and substance abuse.[7]

The US Centers for Disease Control and Prevention (CDC) conducts more than 400,000 health-based interviews annually.[8] Established in 1984, the Behavioral Risk Factor Surveillance System (BRFSS) is the largest continuous survey of its kind in the world. An exhaustive study, *Long-Term Physical Health Consequences of Adverse Childhood Experiences*, examined four years of BRFSS data from over 50,000 adults.[9] The CDC reports that up to 21 million cases of depression and 1.9 million cases of heart disease could have been avoided if critical strategies to prevent ACEs had been implemented.[10]

Sadly, ACEs are all too common. Research shows that 61 per cent of adults have experienced at least one type of ACE, and nearly one in six report they have experienced four or more types of ACEs.[11] ACEs are costly as well, with the economic and social burden to families, communities and society totaling hundreds of billions of dollars each year.[12]

Are we literally "born into" trauma? Otto Rank (1884–1939), an Austrian psychoanalyst and protégé of Sigmund Freud, believed that the birth process is the source of all human anxiety, arguing that we go from a blissful state in the womb to the harsh reality of physical separation.[13] In contrast, contemporary science acknowledges that an expectant mother's exposure to stress can have a profound influence on the unborn child, potentially leading to a host of physical and emotional health outcomes later in life.[14]

In *Windows to the Womb*, psychologist David B. Chamberlain recounts extraordinary case studies of his patients' womb and birth-trauma memories.[15] While under hypnosis, patients were able to access vivid recollections of their gestation period, including their mother's emotional states, the family environment and the details of their own birth.

Psychoneuroimmunology is the study of the interactions between the mind, the nervous system and the immune system, and the science behind how stress and negative emotions can greatly strain our health and wellbeing.[16]

Janice Kiecolt-Glaser, psychologist and professor, addresses how stress and depression affect our immunity. She writes, "We have learned that distress can slow wound healing, diminish the strength of immune responses to vaccines, enhance susceptibility to infectious agents, and reactivate latent viruses."[17]

I spoke with Shamini Jain, psychologist, scientist and Founder and CEO of the Consciousness and Healing Initiative (CHI). Dr. Jain summed up the important principles of this relatively new and growing field. "Psychoneuroimmunology serves as a bridge to not only understand how our emotions affect our health, but how our environment affects our health through our emotional responses," she stated. "Psychoneuroimmunology helps us understand how early childhood trauma perpetuates health disadvantages by creating a set-point in the body that can lead to increased inflammation and therefore increased disease risk."

Inherited trauma may live in our very genes. The term "epigenetics" relates to non-genetic influences that can modify the expression of our genes. Epigenetic research is helping to transform behavioral science by identifying how gene modifications can determine our behaviors and shape our responses to stress.[18] Scientists are studying the transfer of PTSD symptoms and other health problems passed down from first-generation trauma survivors, including combat veterans, refugee families and Holocaust survivors, to their children and to future generations.[19] In a compelling investigation, researchers found, "There is now converging evidence supporting the idea that offspring are affected by parental trauma exposures occurring before their birth, and possibly even prior to their conception."[20]

Ongoing studies in ACEs, psychoneuroimmunology and epigenetics are changing healthcare in significant ways. This new science on the nature of trauma powerfully validates the connections that medical intuitives consistently discern.

Trauma and Healing Traditions

Through leading-edge science we are learning more about how our emotions and our physical health are linked. This concept is not new; it is rooted in ancient healing traditions. The following are only a few examples of the great diversity of energy-based traditional practices.

Traditional Chinese Medicine (TCM) correlates emotions to specific organs, such as anger with the liver, fear with the kidneys and sadness with the heart and lungs.[21] Emotional stress is considered a potent contributor to physical illness by creating a disruption in the flow of vital life force energy, or *qi*.[22]

Shamanism is a widely used term that refers to indigenous spiritual customs from all over the world. Traumatic events are believed to create "soul loss," in which a portion of the person's soul or spirit dissociates from the body.[23] A shamanic practitioner undertakes a spiritual journey to the ancestral or spirit realms to retrieve and help reintegrate these energies.

Past life regression therapy is based on the Hindu philosophy of reincarnation – the belief that a soul may return in a new physical form across many lifetimes. Hypnotic regression is intended to review disturbing incidents in past lives in order to bring awareness to present health issues. Although considered controversial in mainstream mental healthcare, licensed psychotherapists may use these techniques to support the treatment of phobias and other psychological disorders.[24]

Energy healing practices focus on clearing energetic blocks in the biofield believed to be caused by the effects of emotional and physical distress.[25] Practitioners may *feel* for blockages by using light physical touch or by holding their hands a few inches away from the body. Some modalities employ sound frequencies such as tuning forks, gongs and vocal toning.

One of my favorite quotes opens this chapter. Dr. Dean Ornish elegantly states, "Awareness is the first step in healing."[26] As pointed out in Chapter 2, medical intuition is not a direct healing method in itself. However, a qualified medical intuitive can help to raise awareness by identifying the origins of energetic damage in:

- childhood, teenage and adult traumatic life events
- in-utero and birth experiences
- passed-down ancestral epigenetics
- emotions held in organs and body systems
- information stored in past life memories
- energetic blockages affecting the biofield.

As science continues to investigate methods that are as old as humankind itself, the medical world has the opportunity to integrate a broader understanding of trauma. Perhaps we can look forward to a time when healthcare will come full circle, incorporating modern science with ancient spiritual wisdom.

Empowering Permission for Wellness

I have observed that some clients' healing processes are slow or difficult, while others make faster, sometimes even miraculous, recoveries. It's reasonable to wonder why some people heal quickly, others heal more slowly and some not at all. What could be blocking the ability to heal?

Within a session, a trained medical intuitive can measure a client's *permission for wellness*. This evaluation is a "snapshot" of a client's current level of energetic allowance for, or resistance to,

ESSENTIALS OF MEDICAL INTUITION

health and wellbeing. Our levels of permission for wellness are not due to any conscious thought or intention – we all want to heal. Permission levels can be affected by our physical, mental, emotional and spiritual energetic states.

Levels of permission for wellness can also change during a session. You read an example of this potential in Claudia's story in Chapter 1. When Claudia heard what her body wanted her to know regarding the root cause of the tendinitis, her permission for wellness increased. Several days later, she reported that her physical and emotional pain had resolved.

An example of how a low permission for wellness can affect healing is demonstrated in Jerry's story.[27]

CASE STUDY: JERRY

Jerry had a history of back pain, which led to issues with depression. He described the pain as being there as long as he could remember. He had no memory of when it began or a particular incident that could have caused it. Though Jerry had found help through surgery, yoga and antidepressant medication, his level of permission for wellness and relief still looked quite low. Jerry's spine showed me the extent of the physical impairment on his skeletal, nervous and muscular systems. It also showed me years of stored emotional confusion, grief and anger.

I saw that the original injury had occurred when Jerry was just a toddler. On a trip to the supermarket, his mother wanted to give him a special treat of a ride on a mechanical rocking horse, located outside the market's front door. She hoisted him up onto the saddle and tied the strap around his waist. After feeding coins into the slot, the horse started up with a strong jerk. Frightened, Jerry felt the strap give way and he tumbled off the saddle toward the ground. In the fall, his back hit the edge of the concrete slab where the metal horse was welded, injuring his spine. Assuming the little boy's tears were only from the fear and surprise of the fall, unfortunately his injury was overlooked by his mother. Despite Jerry's complaints of pain as he grew up, his concerns were minimized by his doctors and his family. The spinal injury was left untreated until Jerry was ten years old, at which point the pain was so severe that he could not participate in school sports.

Jerry's low permission for wellness reflected the emotional effects of his childhood attempts to explain his constant pain and discomfort. Powerful feelings of frustration and fear were being stored in his back, which appeared to be a major factor in the expression of both his physical condition and his struggles with depression.

As I explained to Jerry what his body was showing me, I noticed his permission for wellness level beginning to rise. His body suggested options to address pain reduction and inflammation, including modalities he hadn't yet considered. Until that point, much of Jerry's daily energy was being used in resistance to his chronic back pain, which further triggered the stored emotions, creating a very debilitating situation. With this session, Jerry was able to put a time, place, and perhaps most importantly, a validation of his life-changing traumatic injury.

Simply put, his own body held all the information he needed to find a deeper understanding of his health and gain a greater level of permission for wellness. After the session, Jerry felt that he was able to begin the process of forgiving himself, his family and his own body.

JOURNAL EXERCISE

Think about a recent health issue. If you were able to have a conversation with your body to find out what it wanted and needed, how do you think your own permission for wellness might have increased?

The Soul's Path

Because both overt and subtle traumatic circumstances are so pervasive in our lives, you may be wondering why we would hold on to any of its effects in our energy. There are as many answers to that question as there are people in the world. As I am not a licensed mental healthcare professional, I do not give psychological advice. As a medical intuitive, I can detect how energetic damage may have limited a client's energy, what may be slowing or stopping the healing process, and the potential next steps in their healing journey.

In my experience, the most essential information that can be gained for exploration, discovery and change is contained in the answers to these questions:

- *Why did this issue manifest?*
- *What can one learn from it?*
- *How can one heal in body, mind and spirit?*

This pivotal inquiry is designed to support the healing process, and helps us to align with our inner guidance and our body's wisdom.

Over my years in practice, I have developed a spiritual perspective about trauma that informs every medical intuitive session I am privileged to give. Every trauma contains our most fundamental life lessons. When we become aware of this meaningful aspect of trauma, we can begin to look inward for insights that help illuminate our soul's path. From this place, the deepest healing can begin.

CHAPTER 8
OUR MARVELOUS META-SENSES

When you reach the end of what you should know, you will
be at the beginning of what you should sense.

Kahlil Gibran

New research is setting the standard for understanding the value of intuition and its relevance to our lives.[1] Intuitive development is encouraged for creative problem-solving and effective business management.[2] The US military funds training to maximize a soldier's "sixth sense," split-second decision-making in combat.[3] Universities and colleges are offering degrees in spirituality and health studies based on nonlocal and intuitive concepts.[4] As we have seen in Chapter 4, modern medicine acknowledges the benefits of practitioner intuition. It seems that intuition is now being taken seriously at the highest levels of education, business, healthcare and government.

But what does the average person believe about intuition? According to a Pew Research Center study, approximately six in ten Americans accept one or more "new age" beliefs, which includes various types of intuition.[5] These beliefs are not replacing their traditional religious convictions. The research found that 61 per cent of Christians ascribe to new age ideas alongside their religious beliefs, with no apparent conflict.

A recent study from the Institute of Noetic Sciences (IONS) examined the prevalence of beliefs in "exceptional human experiences," including clairvoyance, claircognizance and other meta-sensory states.[6] While 94 per cent of the public was shown to believe in intuition, the research surprisingly confirmed that 93.2 per cent of scientists and engineers endorsed it as well. One might think that these two professions would be sensitive to the stigma associated with intuition or to the flouting of scientific norms.

It's best to not make assumptions too quickly. A pioneering survey in the journal *New Scientist* asked more than 1,500 readers, the majority of which were working scientists, if they considered "extrasensory perception" (ESP) to be real or fiction. Nearly 70 per cent believed ESP to be either established fact or highly probable, while 88 per cent thought that ESP was worthy of scientific investigation.[7] Another survey of 1,100 US college professors and academics from the natural sciences, social sciences, arts and humanities, found that 55–77 per cent accepted ESP as fact or at least as a likely possibility.[8]

In learning to acknowledge our innate relationship to intuition, we are evolving from the mechanistic view that has been in play for most of the last century, to a broader perspective that can validate and harness intuition for the betterment of humanity.

Scientific Minds Want to Know ...

From the mid-19th century through the early 20th century, an explosion of interest in the paranormal swept Europe and the US, captivating millions of people.

In 1882, some of the most respected British scientists and scholars of the day founded the Society for Psychical Research (SPR) to investigate the "debatable phenomena" of intuitive practices.[9] The American Society for Psychical Research (ASPR) was founded in 1885 and led by psychologist William James. Physiologist and Nobel Prize-winner Charles Richet established an additional society in France. In all, more than 14 associated groups sprang up across Europe, the US and Canada, most of which are still in operation today.

The SPR membership was a veritable who's who of great minds and talents.[10] These included physicists Pierre and Marie Curie, psychoanalysts Carl G. Jung and Sigmund Freud, poet Alfred, Lord Tennyson, author Lewis Carroll, scientific pioneer Sir Oliver Lodge, British prime minister William Gladstone, chemist Sir William Crookes, philosopher and Nobel laureate Henri Bergson, along with hundreds of physicians, scientists, psychologists, writers and artists. In order to root out frauds and validate the genuine articles, they established stringent methods and exacting standards for data collection and analysis. The SPR published important early works, and in 1884 created the *Journal of the Society for Psychical Research*. More than 125 years later, the journal is still in publication.[11]

Scientifically vetted research on intuition in the US dates back to the 1930s, with the experiments of Joseph B. Rhine (1895–1980).[12] Rhine introduced the contemporary terms "parapsychology," "psi," and "ESP," and created the first-of-its-kind Parapsychology Laboratory at Duke University in North Carolina. Correctly assuming that ESP was an extension of normal human perception, Rhine chose ordinary people as subjects rather than professional psychics. A colleague of his, psychologist Karl Zener (1903–1964), developed the famous Zener cards, a deck of 25 cards, each depicting one of five symbols – a circle, a plus sign, three wavy lines, a square or a star. Rhine used the cards in his exhaustive and meticulous investigations into claircognizance, telepathy and precognition. After conducting an astonishing 90,000 trials, he declared ESP to be a repeatable and demonstrable occurrence.[13] The Rhine Research Center in Durham, North Carolina, continues his tradition.

While returning to earth from a moon mission, Apollo-14 astronaut Edgar Mitchell had a profound spiritual realization of universal "oneness." His epiphany led him to establish the Institute of Noetic Sciences (IONS) in 1973. Headquartered in Petaluma, California, IONS promotes focused peer-reviewed research on the nature of reality, spirituality and the human meta-senses.

Developing the Meta-Senses

Intuition is often called our "sixth sense," but intuition itself consists of six individual meta-senses. These intuitive states, known as the *clairs*, expand beyond our familiar five senses of sight, smell, hearing, touch and taste.

When people talk about intuition, it's not uncommon to hear jaw-dropping stories of how it dramatically intervened in a dire situation. More often, though, intuition plays a much subtler role in our lives. As you read through this chapter, you may find that one or more of the meta-senses resonate, and you may recognize them in your own life. Even if you have never experienced any of the *clairs*, you are still in the right place. I will explain how we may use our intuition regularly without even realizing it, and how four of our meta-senses are actually prized in our pragmatic society.

The Clairs

Clairvoyance: Clear Seeing

My left shoulder ached. Several trips to the chiropractor and acupuncturist hadn't helped to reduce the pain. In my busy life, I felt I didn't have time to talk with my body about something that I thought should go away on its own. When I finally set a moment aside to use my clairvoyant skills, I immediately saw my shoulder's rotator cuff area light up, with a very inflamed bursa practically glaring at me! It had been trying to get my attention for weeks. I asked the bursa what it wanted and why it wasn't healing. It told me that I was taking on far too much responsibility and that I needed to "let others do the heavy lifting." A belief that I had been

*holding on to for many years popped into my awareness – "If
I don't do it, it won't get done." My shoulder was telling me
that it was finally time to let go of that old story.*

Clairvoyance, or clear seeing, is the ability to see information
without the use of physical sight.[14] The word itself can conjure
up thoughts of sci-fi X-ray vision, or mysterious, all-knowing
mind readers. People often think that clairvoyance requires
special gifts or talents. Believe it or not, we already have a
strong understanding of intuitive *seeing* in our society. This
skill is commonly referred to as using our "mind's eye," and
is the basis of mental visualization, guided imagery and self-
hypnosis techniques.

Clairvoyance is ideal for assessing the body's anatomy and
physiology. Medical intuitives report perceiving detailed visuals
similar to anatomical drawings, X-rays or MRIs. The biofield's
chakra system and auric field may be visualized as colors,
shapes, symbols or other imagery. Clairvoyant perception is
also used by medical intuitives to review pivotal moments in a
client's life history.

A 2020 exploratory study by IONS examined how a trained
clairvoyant "seer" might observe the effects of an energy healing
session.[15] Seventeen healing arts practitioners were engaged to
give sessions to 190 participants with chronic hand or wrist
pain. During the session, the clairvoyant was asked to identify
and record any alterations in the physical bodies and biofields of
both the participant and the practitioner.

The researchers' analysis of the clairvoyant's notes provided
an excellent description of medical intuition, stating, "Physical
symptoms in the participant can be caused by multiple
etiological origins, including physical, emotional (especially
traumatic), spiritual and energetic."

Remote viewing is another clairvoyant skill used to intuitively
see distant sites, including descriptions and locations of objects,
buildings and even people. Remote viewers have assisted police
in locating crime scenes and finding missing persons.[16]

Most notoriously, remote viewing was developed for a long-running US government program that trained clairvoyant spies to gather intelligence on foreign military installations.

Known as the Star Gate Project, it began in 1972 at the Stanford Research Institute (SRI) in Menlo Park, California. Physicists Hal Puthoff, Russell Targ and Edwin May, who joined in 1975, were charged with designing a series of remote viewing experiments for the Central Intelligence Agency (CIA).[17] Remote viewing research at SRI ran for over 20 years and received $20 million in US government funding.

In the first tests of the skill, researchers randomly chose a nearby location, such as a museum or a park.[18] Sequestered back at the SRI laboratory, a remote viewer was asked to draw or describe the target location using only clairvoyant *sight*. These experiments produced amazingly accurate results. As the investigation progressed, it was found that remote viewers, when given only the geographic coordinates, were able to relay the locations and details of classified military operations all over the world.

The remote viewers were so exceptionally accurate that the scientists began referring to the sessions in terms of how many martinis they needed to recover their composure after what they had just witnessed.[19] An "eight-martini" session was considered extraordinary, indeed.

Though many military personnel were trained in remote viewing, four noted remote viewers – Army Intelligence officer Joe McMoneagle, who received a Legion of Merit award for his contributions, and civilians artist Ingo Swann, retired police commissioner Pat Price and photographer Hella Hammid – all consistently provided "eight-martini" results.

In all, more than a dozen US government military and intelligence agencies worked with remote viewers on hundreds of experiments and missions.[20] Among their many startling successes, the Star Gate Project located top-secret military sites, Chinese atomic bomb tests and the coordinates of an enemy submarine and a downed spy bomber. During the 1991 Gulf

War, SCUD missiles, tunnels and chemical warfare laboratories were detected. Remote viewer Pat Price also offered a critical clue that led to the finding of Patty Hearst during her kidnapping in 1974.[21] The Star Gate Project ended in 1995. In 2017, CIA records were released to the public through the Freedom of Information Act.

Clairvoyance was the cornerstone of a fascinating experiment in "intuitive archeology." In 1979, scientist and author Stephan A. Schwartz assembled a group of scientists and remote viewers, including Hella Hammid from the Star Gate Project, to join him for the Alexandria Project.[22] His aim was to have the intuitives locate the ruins of the ancient city of Alexandria, which lay submerged off the coast of Egypt. Schwartz and his team discovered the sites of many spectacular treasures, including a temple to the goddess Isis, the palace of Cleopatra and the ruins of the famed Lighthouse of Pharos – one of the Seven Wonders of the Ancient World.

Intuitive mental visualization requires only one powerful talent. This magical skill is the use of our imagination. The word "imagination" is derived from *imago*, meaning "image," and *imaginari*, meaning "to picture oneself." If you can picture the faces of your loved ones in your mind, or your pet or even your own front door, you are using the foundation of clairvoyance.

EXERCISE: MY MIND'S EYE

How often do you use your mind's eye? Do you visualize your to-do list or daily tasks before you sit down to work? When you think about what you'd like to eat, do you get a visual image in your mind of the food you plan to enjoy? When you think about your loved ones, do you also see a picture of them in your mind's eye?

> **Journal Practice:** Notice how you use your mind's eye in your day. Consider ways to practice strengthening this skill of visualization, such as intentionally picturing the face of someone you love or imagining a beautiful landscape. What are some other ways you could use your imagination to practice *seeing* in your mind's eye?

Clairsentience: Clear Feeling

"Who will volunteer for an energy healing?" asked Louise Hay. About 20 people were crowded into the living room of her apartment in Santa Monica, California. A friend had invited me to this private gathering, and I had no idea what to expect. A pale and fragile-looking young man raised his hand. Louise asked him to lie down on the carpet where she had set out a few sparkling crystals. She asked all of us to close our eyes and use our hands to simply send intentional healing energy to the volunteer. I had never done anything like that before. I closed my eyes and extended my hands. Immediately, I sensed a warm stream of energy flowing from my palms toward the young man, and felt a strong rush of emotion in return. Tears welled up as I silently asked the energy flow to help heal the HIV virus that was weakening his body.

Clairsentience, or clear feeling, is the ability to feel other people's emotional or physical information in our own emotions or physical body. We refer to this connection as "compassion" or "empathy." Empathy helps us to develop strong emotional bonds and deepens communication and understanding.

Many clairsentients report feelings of worry or concern on behalf of a friend or loved one, which can appear for no logical reason, but may later turn out to be justified. Obstetrician Larry Kincheloe relayed one such memorable episode.[23]

> While at home on a weekend, Dr. Kincheloe was notified that one of his patients went into early labor, but that delivery was not expected for several hours. He immediately felt an overwhelming sense that something wasn't right. Checking in with his staff, he was told the patient was fine. But the sensation quickly grew. Despite his staff's assurances, Dr. Kincheloe rushed to the hospital. On his arrival, he heard the mother cry out in distress and ran to her labor room just in time to deliver the baby. Curious about his unique experience, he began trusting and acting on his clairsentience.

Practitioners of manual therapies, such as osteopathy, physical therapy, bodywork and massage, report a clairsentient *feeling* in their hands that helps to guide their treatments.[24] Energy healing practitioners may also feel sensations such as heat, cold, pulsing or tingling in their fingers and palms when working with a client's biofield.[25]

Without strong energetic boundaries, however, empathic people may feel overwhelmed, bombarded or weighed down by the emotions of others. Some may even empathically feel other people's physical pains in their own bodies. Those who work in healthcare from a place of caring and concern may find themselves suffering from compassion fatigue.[26]

In my programs, I teach a method of "compassionate neutrality," designed to mitigate the effects of clairsentient overload while still remaining empathetic.

EXERCISE: HOW DO I FEEL?

Do you recognize yourself as clairsentient? Does all of your caring energy go to helping others, leaving you with less time or attention for your own self-care? Can you feel the emotional distress of others? Do you feel like a "soaked sponge" at the end of the day from taking on other people's emotions?

Journal Practice: When you're feeling emotionally overloaded, take a moment to consider whether your feelings belong to you or to someone else. Think about what you can do to help offload emotional burdens with focused self-care such as exercise or meditation.

Claircognizance: Clear Knowing

I nudged the girl who was standing next to me at the cash register where we rang up customer purchases. "See that guy?" I pointed discreetly at a man in a motorcycle jacket who had just walked through the front door of the Bodhi Tree, a renowned spiritual bookstore in Los Angeles. "He's going to the Buddhism section." We watched as he stopped at a display of brightly colored crystals, then headed to the area of the store devoted to books on Buddhism and Eastern spirituality. "And that lady" – a woman who had been perusing a rack of yoga magazines – "is going to the Astrology section." The woman strode purposefully toward the shelves packed with books on astrology. My workmate looked at me and gaped. "How did you know that? You must have seen them come in here before!" "Nope," I shrugged. "I just knew."

Claircognizance, or clear knowing, is the ability to know information without having any prior knowledge. Perhaps the most widely used meta-sense, we call it having a "hunch," a "gut feeling," "mother's intuition" or "women's intuition."[27] The use of gut feelings in the clinical setting has been well studied, as we saw in Chapter 4. Wall Street traders are known for picking stocks on a hunch.[28] If you have ever called on your "parking spot angel" to guide you to a hard-to-find parking space, you may also be using claircognizance.

Telepathy is a type of claircognizance. From *tele*, meaning "distant," and *pathe*, meaning "experience," telepathy is the claircognizant transfer of thoughts from one person to another.[29] One of the most familiar telepathic occurrences is thinking about a friend or loved one, only to find them reaching out to you by email, text or phone soon after. Or perhaps you have contacted someone who said they had just been thinking about you. While people may shrug this off as serendipity or coincidence, telepathy can create these invisible connections.

A favorite topic of psi investigation, there are many interesting studies on telepathic transference. Biologist and researcher Rupert Sheldrake has carried out many such experiments. In a group of studies using randomized phone calls, participants were asked to guess which of four people was telephoning them before they answered the call.[30] The rate of "chance" guesses was calculated at 25 per cent. The combined results showed a remarkable overall success rate of 40 per cent, well above the rate of chance, demonstrating telepathic ability to be a "robust and repeatable" phenomenon. The research was repeated two years later using emails, and returned an even higher success rate of 43–47 per cent.[31]

EXERCISE: I KNOW WHAT I KNOW

How do you use your own intuitive sense of *knowing*? Do you trust it or shrug it off as coincidence? Do you remember a time when you knew something but didn't know how you knew it? Have you used your "inner knowing" to find

---

the perfect parking space or the right opportunity to take? Have you ever awakened from a dream with new insights or knowledge?

Journal Practice: When you notice a sense of *knowing* about a situation or event, write it in your journal and make sure to add the date. On waking, jot down any memorable dreams. These practices can help you to gain a better sense of how often your claircognizance may occur.

Clairaudience: Clear Hearing

"Mom, turn on the radio," a little voice demanded from the backseat. "There's a song I like that's playing." My mother, not giving much thought to the whims of a six-year-old, switched on the radio of our Chevrolet. I had been humming a popular song to myself, which now poured out of the car speakers at exactly where I had been hearing it in my mind. I didn't think this was strange or unusual – I thought everyone could do it.

Clairaudience, or clear hearing, is the ability to hear information without the use of the physical ears. This may be a lesser-known meta-sense, but many intuitives use it regularly. Clairaudience is commonly called our "inner guidance," "inner wisdom," or the "still, small voice" you might hear during contemplation, prayer or meditation.

Clairaudient encounters are described as helpful, informative or even blissful. Clairaudience may sound like guidance speaking in quiet words, music or tones. Some clairaudients claim to hear the voices of spirit guides, ancestors or angels.

There is an important difference between the meta-sense of clairaudience and the "inner voice" of worry and self-doubt. Developing a supportive internal dialogue is an essential skill for mental health and self-growth. But thoughts that are generated by our minds and emotions are not the same as the clairaudient state of tuning in to auditory intuition.

A distinction must also be made between clairaudience and "hearing voices" as a result of mental illness. A study comparing the voice-hearing experiences of self-identified clairaudients with those of patients diagnosed with mental illness found that the clairaudients heard benevolent and positive voices, while the patients heard negative, disruptive voices.[32] Most notably, clairaudients reported they could control the voice hearing by being able to turn it on or off.

EXERCISE: HEARING GUIDANCE

Have you ever intuitively heard your guidance offering you uplifting messages? Have you intuitively heard soothing music, sparkling bells or other sounds while in meditation or contemplation?

Journal Practice: Notice how you differentiate between the voice of negative self-talk and the quiet, loving voice of inner wisdom. Meditation and mindfulness practices are designed to quiet mental chatter and may help you develop a stronger intuitive connection. What other possibilities could you consider to help open your awareness to auditory intuition?

Clairalience: Clear Smelling

Clairalience, or clear smelling, also known as clairolfaction, is the ability to smell a scent when no odor is present, such as your mother's perfume or your grandfather's cigar. A medical intuitive might use this ability to detect a hidden health imbalance. Be aware that smelling unpleasant "phantom" odors may also be related to health issues and should be checked by a medical professional.

Clairgustance: Clear Tasting

Clairgustance, or clear tasting, is the ability to intuitively taste flavors, without putting anything into the mouth. Some people might intuitively taste a favorite flavor from childhood. Clairgustants might also intuitively taste chemicals, drugs or blood, which can help them more accurately discern a health condition.

Combined Meta-Senses

Within a session, a medical intuitive may utilize one meta-sense exclusively or use several meta-senses at a time. Two techniques that incorporate a mix of meta-senses are "psychometry" and "precognition."

Psychometry: The Measure of the Soul

Although the term sounds charmingly antiquated now, psychometry is the ability to receive intuitive information through the physical sense of touch.[33] By holding or touching an object, a psychometrist uses a combination of several *clairs* to glean specific details on the object's history, including where and why it was created, and even who might have owned it.

Holistic healthcare practitioners may also use psychometry when working with a client or patient. A clairsentient *feeling* can be accompanied by *seeing* flashes of clairvoyant imagery, by claircognizant *knowing* – for example, where the practitioner should move their hands next – or by clairaudient *hearing* of a relevant name or date.

Joseph Rodes Buchanan (1814–1899), a physician and professor of physiology, poetically named the skill "the measure of the soul," coined from *psyche*, meaning "soul," and *metron*, "to measure."[34] Dr. Buchanan tested his medical students by having them hold medications concealed in paper to see if the students could identify them using only psychometry. In further trials he used psychometry to determine the histories of natural and manufactured objects.

In 1893, Dr. Buchanan published *Manual of Psychometry: The Dawn of a New Civilization*. Enthusiastic about the possibilities, he wrote, "The discoveries of psychometry will enable us to explore the history of man ... Aye, the mental telescope is now discovered which may pierce the depths of the past and bring us in full view of the grand and tragic passages of ancient history."[35]

Geologist William Denton (1823–1883) conducted thousands of experiments in psychometry.[36] By touching or holding fragments of rocks, he found that psychometrists were able to see, feel and describe a stone's place of origin – from a fiery lava flow to a frozen glacier.

Eighty years after Buchanan published his opus, John Norman Emerson (1917–1978), a highly distinguished archeologist and president of the Canadian Archeology Association, presented his research on a new field he called "intuitive archeology."[37]

Emerson worked closely with his protégé, psychometrist George McMullen (1920–2008).[38] McMullen, who had no training or background in archeology, proved his worth by holding an ancient artifact in his hand and correctly identifying its location, age and other salient facts. Emerson brought him to archeological excavation sites, where McMullen was able to accurately suggest not only where to dig, but exactly what would be found beneath the dirt. Dr. Emerson published several scholarly articles, and helped to develop the framework of intuitive archeology as a discipline. McMullen went on to join the Alexandria Project (*see above*).

Precognition: Reading the Future

There is no meta-sense more associated with the stereotype of the fortune-telling psychic or mystical seer than precognition, or "reading the future." Meaning "foreknowledge," precognition is the intuitive forecast of a potential outcome. The implications of precognitive accuracy hold the possibility of major benefits to commerce, science, medicine, the global economy and more.

Many studies have attempted to nail down the predictive properties of precognition. Premonitions about major catastrophes, such as the sinking of RMS *Titanic*, the Aberfan disaster in Wales, the September 11, 2001 hijackings, floods and other natural disasters, have given scientists much data to sift through.[39] Researchers have even investigated the length between the time an event was predicted and the actual time it took place. Interestingly, they noted that approximately 50 per cent of these predictions occurred within two days, and about 20 per cent took a month or more to transpire.[40]

Studies on the use of precognition in sports betting and the stock market have shown varying levels of success.[41] But some studies have done surprisingly well. One university experiment used a type of precognition called "associative remote viewing" (ARV) to predict the rise and fall of the Dow Jones Industrial Average.[42] Incredibly, the participants' predictions were 100 per cent accurate in 7 out of 7 trials. Stock investments they made based on the results produced a hefty financial windfall for all.

Precognitive warning dreams about health concerns have helped to save people's lives. Greek philosopher Aristotle was convinced of the importance of prescient dreams. He wrote, "The beginnings of diseases and other distempers which are about to visit the body ... must be more evident in the sleeping state."[43]

Patients' dreams that have occurred before the onset of conditions, such as epilepsy, heart disease, kidney failure and cancer, have also helped doctors to hone in on the causes of illness and aid in diagnosis and treatment.[44]

Precognitions which occur while dreaming may include a combination of the following meta-senses.

- Claircognizance: a sense of conviction about the importance of the information; an awareness of actions to be taken.

- Clairvoyance: dream imagery that is more vivid and intense than ordinary dreams; seeing or reading the words of an illness or condition; symbols that are interpreted as relating to health.
- Clairsentience: feelings of emotional dread, threat or menace; experiencing physical symptoms within a dream, such as heat, cold or pain.
- Clairaudience: hearing details or directives about a health issue from a friend, doctor or advisor.

I must inject a word of caution about the use of precognition in healthcare. As we have seen in the effects of the placebo and nocebo responses in Chapter 6, our minds can have a direct influence on our positive or negative health outcomes. Mind–body leaders, such as Quimby, Simonton and Chopra, have shown us the power of our thoughts, beliefs and choices. It has been said that the future is not carved in stone, but written in pencil. I believe it is the ethical and moral responsibility of medical intuitives to support and honor the sacred nature of a client or patient's free will to create their own future.

CHAPTER 9

MEDICAL INTUITION FOR SELF-CARE

There is more wisdom in your body than in your deepest philosophy.

Friedrich Nietzsche

A common thread weaves through all of the sessions I have given, which defines the essence of medical intuition – our bodies have their own awareness and distinct points of view. They have a fear of mortality and a fear of pain and suffering. Very much like small children, they yearn for our reassurance, attention, support and love.

In this chapter, you will have the opportunity to learn some of the foundational techniques of medical intuition for self-healing and self-care. I believe that tapping into our internal "guidance system" is our most important intuitive skill. A good place to begin is by discovering your "Intuitive IQ." No matter where you are on the scale below, remember that you can develop your intuition even further. Consider how you've used your intuition in the past and where intuition might enhance your life now.

Intuitive IQ Self-Test

Answer each question with:
3 points for OFTEN
2 points for SOMETIMES
1 point for NEVER

Points

1. I trust my gut instincts and hunches to help me make decisions. _____

2. I get intuitive hits or flashes of insight that I can't explain. _____

3. I get the answers to my life's questions during meditation, prayer or quiet contemplation. _____

4. I can feel other people's emotions and/or physical pain. _____

5. I have an excellent internal "lie detector." _____

6. I can *sense* the energy of a room or building when I first walk into it. _____

7. People wonder how I make decisions with certainty, even without having complete information. _____

8. I know when someone I care for is in distress, before I am aware of the situation. _____

9. Before a negative event occurs, I have a sense of foreboding or worry. _____

10. Before a positive event occurs, I have a sense of optimism or happiness. _____

11. I have avoided scary or dangerous situations by using my intuition. _____

12. I wake up after sleep with answers to questions I have been thinking about. _____

13. My creative ideas feel as if they come from "somewhere else." _____

14. My intuition communicates in quiet words, phrases or sounds. _____

15. I can *see* intuitive images in my mind's eye. _____

16. Friends and loved ones come to me for emotional support or personal advice. _____

17. I follow up on my hunches, whether or not they seem logical. _____

Total Points _____

Answer Key

17 points: Beginning Intuition

If you answered "Never" to all of the questions, you can still learn to access your intuition. The exercises in this book are designed to help you notice when your intuition sparks, even if only for an instant. Becoming aware of these quick hits can help your intuition to grow.

18–28 points: Developing Intuition

You may be learning to trust your intuition and have already used it to help navigate your life from time to time. Even if your intuition seems like it comes and goes, you can learn to strengthen it to be more reliable and dependable. You're off to a great start!

29–39 points: Expressing Intuition

You are likely to acknowledge your intuitive nature and may feel attuned to your own internal compass. You may be using your intuition to connect with the emotions and experiences of family, close friends or others. You also may be accessing your intuition in your career or life goals, which can give you extra insight to get ahead. Keep paying attention to the messages your intuition brings.

40–51 points: Integrating Intuition

People may wonder about your special intuitive gift! You may have a strong, positive relationship with your intuition and are likely to be using it daily to help guide you through life's decisions. You may also feel a sense of life purpose or mission, perhaps with a focus toward the healing and betterment of humanity.

A WORD OF CAUTION BEFORE YOU BEGIN THE EXERCISES

Developing intuition is a profoundly personal process. As you connect to your intuitive self, the exercises may evoke a range of unexpected feelings, sensations or emotions. This is perfectly normal. Be aware of any insights or enlightening moments that may occur.

Connecting to your intuition may also feel disquieting or bring up physical or emotional discomfort. If you experience any physical or emotional distress during any of the exercises, please stop immediately and take a few deep, calming breaths. Begin again only if and when you are ready. If any exercise feels overwhelming, you are advised to stop and to seek professional care, if appropriate.

It is important to practice in a safe, calm and supportive environment. Go slowly and give yourself all the time you need. Please note that intuitive visualization is not intended to be a substitute for psychological or medical diagnosis and treatment, and it does not replace the services of licensed healthcare providers. Always refer to a licensed healthcare professional for medical or psychological care.

The Language of Imagery

The foundations of medical intuition begin with an understanding of the mind–body connection. As noted in Chapter 6, study after study shows how directed mental imagery can enhance our vitality and ability to heal. Intuitive visualization is a powerful way to forge a relationship between our minds and our bodies.

If you have any difficulty visualizing, don't worry – just "get what you get." Any intuitive information is welcome.

Remember, the only skill you need to access your intuition is your own imagination. Be gentle with yourself as you practice, and most of all, have fun!

There are three reasons that I offer these self-healing visualization exercises:

- Nurses asked me for energetic tools to help them maintain resilience while working in the high-pressure hospital environment.
- Clients asked me how to manage their own energy to help them navigate their personal healing journeys.
- My students wanted useful resources to recommend to their clients and patients.

To get started, here is a simple exercise to illustrate how our bodies speak the language of imagery. Read through the exercise first and then practice with your eyes closed. Go slowly and see what happens.

EXERCISE: CAN MY MIND AFFECT MY BODY?

Start by asking your body to produce saliva. Don't give it a lot of thought – just see what it takes to create some saliva in your mouth. Notice if you are moving your tongue or mouth as you try. Does it take a lot of effort to create a little saliva?

Now, close your eyes and take a deep, relaxing breath in and out. Then, breathe normally.

In your mind's eye, imagine you're holding a large, ripe, juicy lemon in your hand. Imagine you can feel the weight and shape of it in your palm. Does it feel heavy or light?

Now, bring the lemon up to your nose and take a deep sniff. Imagine you can smell the fresh, bright lemony scent.

Put your teeth against the skin of the lemon and imagine you can feel the gentle pressure … Then, bite right through the lemon skin.

Taste the sharp, sour tang of the lemon juice filling up your mouth and feel the bitter pulp squish between your teeth. Keep chewing the lemon pulp as the tart, juicy flavor surrounds your tongue and fills up your senses … Take your time.

Notice if you're producing saliva.

Journal Practice: Begin to notice the role your thoughts and emotions might play in how your body feels. Does a positive thought feel physically lighter? Does a negative thought feel heavier? Consider incorporating some mind–body practices into your life, such as meditation, breath work, affirmations or guided imagery. What other mind–body practices could you consider trying?

Energy Hygiene

Good hygiene helps us maintain our physical health. Have you ever thought about the state of your energy hygiene? Most people don't realize this is an area of our health to consider. Energy hygiene techniques are intended to help build energetic resilience and assist you in creating an intuitive bond between body, mind and spirit.

This chapter presents three energy hygiene tools: grounding, shielding and releasing. You will also have the opportunity to learn two self-healing visualizations. People have found these energy tools to be practical, effective and easy to follow. Read slowly through the scripts and practice as you go. You can also have a friend read them aloud to you. Above all, they are designed to be enjoyable.

Grounding: Putting Down Roots

The use of physical grounding, sometimes called "earthing," involves walking barefoot on sand, grass or dirt, or wading in a natural body of water. Earthing mats or pads can be used indoors for rest or sleep. Earthing shows positive benefits for generating greater health and wellbeing.[1]

This first energy hygiene exercise uses intuitive imagery for grounding. To do this, imagine creating a strong connection between your body and the earth. This type of grounding is often used in meditation, guided imagery and in many energy-healing modalities. Energetic grounding can help to lower stress and create a sense of centeredness and calm.

EXERCISE: GROUNDING

Begin by sitting in a comfortable chair with your feet flat on the floor. Close your eyes and take two deep, relaxing breaths in and out. With each exhale, release any physical tension or stress. Then, breathe normally.

In your mind's eye, imagine vine roots or tree roots growing from the soles of your feet, reaching down into the rich earth. These roots allow you to feel the solid stability of the earth. Imagine that you can feel the gentle support of the earth.

Now, locate any physical tension or tiredness in your body. Let that tension or tiredness flow right down your grounding roots, deep into the earth. Imagine that the earth can absorb and transform any tension or tiredness into healing earth energy.

Take a deep breath in, and let it out slowly. When you are ready, open your eyes.

If the sensation of a vine or tree root feels too heavy, try imagining your grounding roots as beams of light, a stream of energy or any image you may prefer.

Shielding: Your Energetic Comfort Zone

Shielding imagery is designed to create a sense of protection, comfort and safety. Shielding can be used with the intention of keeping other people's energies from affecting your own. This energy tool can be useful if you are highly empathic or clairsentient, or for those who work in healthcare or with the public.

EXERCISE: SHIELDING

Begin by sitting in a comfortable chair with your feet flat on the floor. Close your eyes and take two deep, relaxing breaths in and out. With each exhale, release any physical tension or stress. Then, breathe normally.

In your mind's eye, send grounding roots down from the soles of your feet, connecting you solidly to the earth.

Now, imagine that you have a 3ft-thick buffer of protective light all around your body. You may choose any color you like for your buffer. This buffer of light may look fluffy, like cotton candy, cotton balls or clouds, or it may look shimmery and full of sparkles. Imagine it looking exactly as you'd like to visualize it.

Now, imagine you can see right through your buffer into the world around you. In your mind's eye, imagine yourself going through your day with this 3ft-thick buffer all around you. See yourself at your job with your buffer up. How do you interact with people now, and how do they interact with you?

Now imagine a challenging or difficult person in your life — someone who can really "push your buttons." Keep your buffer up, and watch that person doing their difficult thing … Notice how you feel. Does your buffer help you feel calmer and more centered?

Take a deep breath in, and let it out slowly. When you are ready, open your eyes.

Grounding and shielding imagery can be used throughout your day, with your eyes open or closed. Notice how your energy feels after using these two energy hygiene tools. Are you feeling energetically overloaded or do you feel more calm and centered?

One question my students ask is, "Can I hug someone with my shielding buffer up?" Yes, you can. You can even be in a crowded elevator with your buffer up, without bumping into anyone! Why? Energy is based on the power of intention. Wayne Dyer wrote, "You create your thoughts, your thoughts create your intentions, and your intentions create your reality."[2] You can practice using your intention when working with your energy.

Releasing: Managing Your Energy Balance

Releasing is intended to help let go of unwanted energy, such as thoughts, feelings or emotions that may weigh you down with negativity or stress. Releasing techniques are not meant to keep us from experiencing our emotions. Processing our feelings is critical to maintaining mental and emotional health. This energy tool is a simple method designed to help you shift your personal energy in the moment, whenever you choose.

EXERCISE: RELEASING

Begin by sitting in a comfortable chair with your feet flat on the floor. Close your eyes and take two deep, relaxing breaths in and out. With each exhale, release any physical tension or stress. Then, breathe normally.

In your mind's eye, send grounding roots down from the soles of your feet, connecting you solidly to the earth.

Imagine that you have a 3ft-thick buffer of light all around your body.

Now, take a moment to inventory what you may be feeling emotionally right now. Do you notice any stress, worry, sadness, anger or frustration? Perhaps you had a difficult day at your job, a tough conversation with a loved one, or a concern about finances or health.

Notice any feelings, thoughts or emotions that you would like to release. See if you can identify where those feelings might be located in your body.

In your mind's eye, imagine a large translucent soap bubble floating in front of you at eye level. This soap bubble can hold all of the cares, worries, concerns and emotions that you identified.

Now, imagine that you can pull all of those feelings out of your energy and put them directly into the center of the soap bubble. This soap bubble can expand as big as you need it to be. Take your time and fill it up.

When the soap bubble is full, imagine a big WHOOSH of air sending it high into the sky. In your mind's eye, see it getting smaller and smaller as it floats higher and higher.

When it gets so small that you can barely see it, imagine it POP! Everything you put into the soap bubble turns into golden sparkles in the sunlight and simply dissolves.

Now, think of a positive word, like PEACE, CALM or RELEASE. Take a deep breath in, and, as you breathe out, say that positive word either to yourself or out loud. Let the energy of the word fill your mind, heart and spirit.

When you are ready, open your eyes.

I suggest incorporating grounding, shielding and releasing into your day. Feeling a bit energetically off-kilter? Send down your grounding roots. Feeling overwhelmed by the energy of others? Shield your energy with a buffer. Dealing with a stressful to-do list? Release any unwanted energy into a soap bubble. These intentional energy hygiene practices can help you learn how to manage and balance your own energy, in every moment of every day.

Your Body's Wisdom: A Conversation for Self-Healing

Intuitive communication can allow us to listen to and trust the messages our bodies give us. In this exercise, you will have the opportunity to create an intentional and meaningful conversation with your own body. Because this is a deeper guided meditation, a script is not included here. Please visit the "Guided Meditations" page at The Practical Path website, www.thepracticalpath.com/guided-meditations. Choose the guided meditation titled *Your Body's Wisdom*.

Your Healing Toolkit

In Chapter 6, I related my healing story of shrinking a tumor by visualizing a cheerful scrub brush and giggling soap bubbles dissolving it away. Imagery for self-healing is well established in the scientific literature and has been used successfully for pain reduction, positive surgery outcomes and more.[3] Best of all, imagery is fun and easy to use.

There are many resources for healing visualizations. Shakti Gawain's *Creative Visualization*, written in 1978, became an instant classic and helped to fuel worldwide interest in mind–body imagery.[4] The book *How Your Mind Can Heal Your Body* by scientist and author David R. Hamilton offers a wealth of visualizations designed for many physical conditions.[5] Kaiser Permanente and other hospital networks offer Belleruth Naparstek's guided imagery meditations, Health Journeys.[6]

Some of my favorite healing tools include imagining a miniature golden vacuum cleaner to remove anything unwanted; cool air or refreshing water to bring down inflammation; and special salves and tonics to assist the body's natural healing ability. Color and light are also wonderful healing tools. Try green for healthy growth, pink for love energy, orange for vibrancy, and blue for calming.

Positive affirmations are excellent additions to your healing toolkit. One of the most famous affirmations, "Every day, in every way, I am getting better and better," was created by Émile Coué (1857–1926), a French psychologist.[7] Affirmations can help to align our bodies and minds for vibrant health and wellbeing.

In the next exercise, you can begin to create your own customized imagery toolkit for self-healing and self-care. Start by choosing a part of your body to work with. You will then imagine a set of energetic healing tools. There is no limit to the kind of imagery you can use. Be creative! However, please avoid negative visuals. If your physical body would not like it, do not use it.

As you use your healing toolkit, please be in a calm and positive frame of mind, and visualize the body issue healing as you work.

EXERCISE: CREATE YOUR HEALING TOOLKIT

Begin by sitting in a comfortable chair with your feet flat on the floor. Close your eyes and take two deep, relaxing breaths in and out. With each exhale, release any physical tension or stress. Then, breathe normally.

In your mind's eye, send grounding roots down from the soles of your feet, connecting you solidly to the earth.

Imagine you have a 3ft-thick buffer of light all around your body.

In your mind's eye, imagine you are looking at a part of your body that you'd like to help heal.

Now, you will create a healing tool. As you use it, imagine that you can see this part of your body healing perfectly. If one healing tool doesn't work the way you want it to, try another. Use as many healing tools as you like.

And now, give your body a positive affirmation.

Finally, imagine filling this part of your body with golden light and see it glow. Expand the golden light outward to fill your whole body – all the way up to the top of your head and all the way down to the tips of your toes.

Take a deep breath in, and let it out slowly. When you are ready, open your eyes.

Audio recordings for some of the exercises in this chapter are available on the "Guided Meditations" page at www.thepracticalpath.com/guided-meditations. If you would like further instruction on how to use intuition and energy tools, please visit the website for information on programs and workshops.

CHAPTER 10

SEEING INTO THE FUTURE OF HEALTHCARE

Every now and then a man's mind is stretched by a new idea or sensation, and never shrinks back to its former dimensions.

Oliver Wendell Holmes, Sr.

People who seek out professional medical intuitives have often "been through the mill" of mainstream medicine. Many report having seen dozens of doctors and have taken a multitude of tests. Their health issues have been missed, minimized, over- or undertreated or even ignored. Some have been devastated to learn from their doctors that there were no further options for relief. Even when turning to the holistic healing arts, which can hold so much potential and hope, people may spend thousands of dollars on endless options. These clients tell me they have "tried everything and nothing has worked," and I believe them.

This situation does not occur because practitioners have failed. It is because the lens through which they are trained to look does not, and cannot, deliver the intuitive 360-degree view. A practitioner's own body of knowledge – the optics through which they must view every issue – may be the very thing that keeps them from most effectively helping their patient or client.

Medical intuition is a different kind of lens. It offers a direct line of communication and inquiry from the broadest point of view down to the minutiae of our cells. This perspective incorporates the wonder of our bodies, the limitless power of our minds, our unique life histories, and the boundless beauty of the human spirit. These intrinsic aspects are meant to work in concert to support healing in the physical, emotional, mental, spiritual and energetic realms.

A New Definition of Health

The World Health Organization (WHO) defines "health" as, "A state of complete physical, mental and social wellbeing and not merely the absence of disease or infirmity."[1] The National Center for Complementary and Integrative Health (NCCIH) recently created a new definition of whole-person health as, "supporting the health and wellbeing of each person across multiple domains – biological, behavioral, social, and environmental."[2]

According to Helene Langevin, physician and Director of the NCCIH, viewing health from the biomedical standpoint of "pieces and parts" is no longer sustainable, and scientific inquiry, though crucial, is not enough. For people to thrive and not merely survive, she argues that we must "'reassemble' the pieces and parts of health and see the whole person."[3]

These relatively new definitions of health represent a pivotal shift in the Western medicine mindset. It is wonderful to see conventional medicine broadening its point of view, rather than focusing only on the diagnosis and treatment of symptoms and diseases. For medical intuitives, these expanded definitions have existed at the foundation of our work under the rubrics of "body" and "mind." So, how does "spirit" fit into the model of whole-person health?

A 2020 article in *Global Advances in Health and Medicine* proposed that whole-person health must take into account the nonlocal, transcendent aspects of human awareness.[4] It is time for medicine to recognize and integrate the intuitive and spiritual side of wellness. I will respectfully add one more definition to help push the envelope a bit further. Let's also define health as our spiritual natures working in harmony with our minds and bodies.

When I had the idea to write this book, I knew I wanted to feature some of the world leaders in intuitive, holistic healthcare. I was honored to speak with three trailblazers: Dr. Gladys T. McGarey, Dr. Lucia Thornton and Dr. Larry Dossey.

The Physician Within

An internationally recognized pioneer of integrative health, physician Gladys T. McGarey is affectionately known as the Mother of Holistic Medicine. Dr. McGarey is co-founder of both the American Holistic Medical Association and the Academy of Parapsychology and Medicine. Her organization, The Foundation for Living Medicine, is dedicated to transforming the current disease-based model of healthcare to one that embraces an individual's journey to wholeness.[5] As of this writing, she is a formidable force at the remarkable age of 100.

Dr. McGarey describes her philosophy as an approach created to consciously empower the "physician within" each of us. "Medical intuition is vital to the practice of medicine," she asserts. "Every physician who truly wants to practice what I call Living Medicine must have the doctor within them access the doctor within each patient. That connection is medical intuition."

Dr. McGarey feels the intuitive process truly honors a patient's reality. "A medical intuitive does not impose their prejudices onto the person they're working with. That is what MDs do all the time," she says. Instead, a skilled medical intuitive "listens to the inner doctor of the patient, and can then begin to get a true understanding."

On the potential of incorporating medical intuition into the clinical setting, Dr. McGarey states, "The possibilities are huge. Intuition is the only way medicine will progress. Unless we can accept this, we will be working only with diseases and pain and not with the patient themselves." Dr. McGarey believes the physician's focus must be on "Life and love – that is what healing is about."

The Heart and Spirit of Caring

Lucia Thornton, Doctor of Theology and nurse, holds a vision for a new spirit of compassionate, sustainable healthcare. Her book, *Whole Person Caring: An Interprofessional Model for Healing and Wellness*, presents a framework for nurturing healthcare environments that emphasize a spiritual approach. She describes "Whole Person Caring" as "bringing heart and soul back into our lives and work, and advocating for a healthcare system that does the same."[6]

Dr. Thornton's nursing and teaching career spans more than 40 years. She has served as past president of the American Holistic Nurses Association (AHNA) and board chair of the Academy of Integrative Health & Medicine (AIHM).

As a nurse, Lucia Thornton had many intuitive encounters. "I would know when things were going to happen before they would happen," she says. A memorable incident occurred one evening while she was at work in the Intensive Care Unit (ICU). A patient was admitted who had suffered a massive stroke. Brain scans showed no response, and the family was sent home with the agonizing task of deciding whether or not to prolong the life of their loved one.

She intuitively sensed the patient's presence was "still there," even though there was no medical evidence. She began speaking quietly to the patient with empathy and compassion. Inexplicably, a single tear slowly slid down the patient's cheek. Through the rest of her shift, she continued to convey gentle words of encouragement and hope. The next morning the patient's eyes opened. Two weeks later, the patient was discharged from the hospital. This experience was the ultimate test of trusting her intuition, and it generated a profound shift in her awareness.

"It is so important for medicine to begin to understand that we are spiritual beings and not just biomedical entities," Dr.

Thornton says. "Once we recognize this, we will have a context in which intuition makes sense. Until then, everything in our medical system will only be focused on the physical. This narrow point of view is what has thrown the entire medical model out of balance." She feels it is critical to include this topic in medical and nursing school curricula.

Her concepts make economic sense, as well. Hospital implementations of Dr. Thornton's program are noted for raising nurse retention rates to well above the national average, saving hospitals millions of dollars in staff turnover. Her program has achieved industry recognition for increased patient and staff satisfaction, and excellence in patient care.[7]

Dr. Thornton holds a vision for healthcare as a sacred practice that honors our essence, with self-care, self-healing and self-compassion. "Redefining who we are as spiritual beings creates the underpinnings for a new paradigm of health going forward," Dr. Thornton states. "This broader view can influence both our research and our practices."

A New Era of Medicine

Physician and author Larry Dossey travels the world talking to medical professionals about integrating intuitive, nonlocal consciousness concepts into healthcare. In his visionary book, *Reinventing Medicine: Beyond Mind-Body to a New Era of Healing*, Dr. Dossey divides modern medicine into three eras.[8] Era I, dating from the mid-19th through the early 20th centuries, represented the dawn of scientific medical methods and a predominantly mechanistic view of the human body. Era II, beginning in the mid-20th century, brought new theories of how the mind and emotions influence physical health – what we now call mind–body medicine. Dr. Dossey sees medicine rapidly approaching Era III, a future that blends current medicine with intuitive energy-based practices, and medical intuition in particular.

"Medical intuition isn't logical. It isn't rational. It's a kind of *knowing* that, in spite of our logical inclinations, bursts through," Dr. Dossey says. "A lot of people who think that they're using their intuition are playing around in the shallow end of the pool. They may be pointing in the right direction, but I don't think it goes far enough."

Dr. Dossey firmly believes that incorporating medical intuition into the medical school curriculum is critical to the transition into Era III medicine. "Era III involves action – having a concrete plan and goal for a real change. There's nothing wrong with attention to the physical in medical training," he states, but feels that education falls short when only the physical is addressed.

"Medical intuition has been around for a long time, but it hasn't been honored," Dr. Dossey says. He points out that medical intuitives generally work outside of the formal healthcare structure, and that physicians who use medical intuition find it difficult to discuss their experiences with colleagues. It is his belief that we can, and should, do better.

The good news is that Dr. Dossey finds that most healthcare providers are very receptive to the need for medical intuition, but there are challenges in helping to break through barriers. "More evidence-based science would help," he suggests. "We have to take a philosophical look backwards. Sometimes it takes decades for research to achieve an effect. If medicine is famous for one thing, it's honoring tradition. And radical change is like pulling teeth." Dr. Dossey stresses there are now numerous peer-reviewed studies providing incontrovertible evidence for nonlocal consciousness as applied in healthcare.[9]

As medicine begins to embrace the concepts of integrative health, Dr. Dossey remains hopeful, but he cautions that these models must expand to add intuitive and consciousness education. "Some integrative practitioners think that elaborating on the current worldview by introducing things like exercise, diet and better nutrition is 'new medicine.' They don't seem to get it," he says. "And, in that sense, they're stuck in the old paradigm without realizing it."

So what might Dr. Dossey's idea for a future of medicine that includes medical intuition really look like?

A Flash of Insight vs. a Complete Medical Intuitive Assessment

Practitioners from many disciplines are familiar with the experience of intuitive hits, or flashes of insight – random moments of clarity. Although intuitive flashes can be very illuminating, they can also be unpredictable in how they appear, unrepeatable on demand and even incomplete. The differences between an intuitive flash and a comprehensive medical intuitive assessment are significant. Medical intuition is intended to be accessible, repeatable and complete in scope and depth of detail. The best way for me to explain this is with an example from my early career as an energy healing practitioner, compared to how I work today as a medical intuitive.

CASE STUDY: A FLASH OF INSIGHT

Ray came to see me with a painful and swollen knuckle on his left-hand ring finger. During the energy healing session, I received an intuitive flash of insight that his knuckle was storing an overwhelming sense of grief. His ring finger looked like it was ready to cry!

When I mentioned this to Ray, he told me that a few days earlier, a serious relationship had ended with a woman who he felt was "the one." Ray was devastated. However, the thought that he might lose her as a friend was even more painful, so he kept his feelings quietly on the inside.

In another flash of insight, I pointed out to Ray that these unexpressed emotions were being held precisely in the place where a wedding band would have gone – on the ring finger of his left hand. Ray understood that his body was telling him to process his pent-up grief and sadness.

This case is an excellent example of how the body can store emotional energy and how a practitioner may receive intuitive flashes. But what else could I have done for Ray if I had conducted a medical intuitive session first?

Ray 2.0 with a Medical Intuitive Assessment

Ray, a massage therapist, uses his hands to earn his living. With medical intuition, I begin by intuitively scanning his hand and knuckle to detect any potential physical damage that might need medical attention.

I assess if the injury might create an area of weakness that could hinder his vocation, and review options that may help him prevent any further damage. I can perceive the impact of the physical pain and stress. I can also conduct an intuitive scan of his entire body and repeat the in-depth scanning technique as needed.

Next, I can intuitively discern choices and recommendations from his body's own perspective designed to help him create a path to healing. This includes referring Ray to a range of appropriate health professionals and, most importantly, to his licensed primary care provider before he makes any changes to his current health routine.

In scanning his biofield, what else might I see for Ray? Regarding his emotional grief and pain, I can identify energetic damage that may be held in his biofield (*see* Chapter 7). I can take a look at his fourth chakra, which represents the ability to both give and receive love. I may also evaluate his second chakra, which governs emotional balance and intimacy, and his third chakra, the center of self-esteem. The medical intuitive assessment can reveal how crucial moments in Ray's life story may have led him to give his heart to someone who could not love him in the way he truly deserved.

Medical intuition is designed to help me evaluate the best opportunities for Ray to release any blocked energy, so that he can be more open to finding true partnership. It can lead me directly to the solutions that may give him the most beneficial support, whether or not a particular modality is part of my personal body of knowledge. For Ray, I can observe if somatic therapies, journaling or the help of a licensed counselor or psychologist might be beneficial. I might also review various stress reduction techniques, such as meditation, movement or spending time in nature. I can even determine if my own energy-healing modality would be the right match for Ray.

Finally, the medical intuitive session can help Ray understand what may be affecting permission for wellness in his body and biofield (*see* Chapter 7). In short, medical intuition can offer Ray relevant and meaningful information intended to help him mend both his hand and his heart.

The Doctor of the Future

In Chapter 5, you learned how doctors are working side by side with medical intuitives to achieve remarkable health successes for their patients. You have also read data revealing that a majority of people trust their medical intuitives at least as much as they trust their primary care providers.

Let's take a moment to imagine a visit with the doctor of the future. If you are a licensed healthcare provider, consider whether you are ready to include medical intuition in your practice. If you are a patient or client, consider if this is the kind of care you would like to receive from your doctor.

DOCTOR AS MEDICAL INTUITIVE

First, imagine that your patients are not putting off their appointments until a health disaster strikes! They know medical intuition can give you a broader understanding of their wellness concerns, so they feel heard and respected. You've seen how this can raise compliance and allow them to become a partner in their own healing journey.[10] You also find that medical intuition can help you fine-tune and streamline your care plans, tests and treatments to your patients' individual needs. Medical intuition offers the very opposite of the cookie-cutter approach they are likely to have experienced with prior practitioners.

You know that a medical intuitive assessment can provide you with fast and pertinent information. Your examination process always includes a medical intuitive scan, either by conducting it yourself before, during or after the appointment, or by interacting directly with your medical intuitive team member, or by ordering a referral to a qualified medical intuitive consultant.

With medical intuition, you can review hidden factors that may be contributing to health issues, including vital insights into why a patient may not be healing, despite best efforts.[11] Most critically, you can discover what may be driving their wellness challenges at the core level by intuitively assessing life stressors, energetic damage and permission for wellness (see Chapter 7).

Medical intuition gives you, the licensed practitioner, the opportunity to create a patient-centered, whole-person roadmap intended to help your patients achieve full-spectrum wellbeing.

Does this sound like a fantasy? It doesn't have to. Medical intuition can be scaled from an Emergency Room encounter to a full office visit. I believe that medical intuitives should be on staff at every clinic and hospital, and that medical intuition should be taught as an essential part of healthcare training.

What's Next for Medical Intuition?

Daniel H. Pink, author of *A Whole New Mind: Why Right-Brainers Will Rule the Future*, wrote, "The future belongs to a very different kind of person with a very different kind of mind."[12] He points to creative and holistic "right-brain" thinkers whose abilities will "mark the fault line between who gets ahead and who gets left behind." Medical intuitives are known for being innovative and creative thinkers, and are eager to be accepted and respected by modern medicine.

Guidelines for best practices are imperative to elevate the field. Of professional medical intuitives surveyed, 76 per cent indicated a strong interest in a national organization to advance vetting, research and outreach for medical intuition.[13] At this time, discussions are ongoing for the formation of a US organization to provide professional standards of practice and codes of ethical conduct, and to promote medical intuition as a recognized skill in clinical medicine and in professional private practice.

This is the starting point for a fundamental systems change in healthcare. "Systems change" is defined as: "An intentional process designed to alter the status quo by shifting the function or structure of an identified system with purposeful interventions. It is a journey which can require a radical change in people's attitudes as well as in the ways people work."[14]

Medical intuition is nothing less than a paradigm-shifting, transformational systems change for the healthcare of tomorrow. Imagine what medical intuition can bring to the frontlines of critical health environments in the Emergency Room and ICU, to scientific and medical research, to the development of new healthcare technologies, to integrative health education, and to a deeper understanding of the root causes of illness and wellness.

Here's the bottom line: medical intuitives are already working in these areas every day. Medical intuition has no limitations in terms of what can be perceived, and its wider benefits to health and science are as yet untapped.

There is no one-size-fits-all for wellbeing. Our bodies and energetic systems are vast and deep, and everyone's story is wholly unique. Ultimately, medical intuition can help us understand the multifaceted nature of who we are, how we are and why we are. It is my hope and wish that medical intuition helps to shed a ray of light on how we can create a more profound and permanent opportunity for healing in body, mind and spirit.

ACKNOWLEDGMENTS

Over the past year, as I sat down at my computer to write this book, I felt like I was diving into a deep blue ocean. Occasionally, I would look up to see the rest of the world buzzing away above the surface. Up there, our world was dealing with a global pandemic, political and social upheaval, and worsening climate crises. In 2021, it is crystal-clear how much humanity, and our planet, is in need of intuitive, holistic healing. I wish everyone health and renewal through truly challenging times.

Though writing a book may feel like a solitary experience, in reality it takes the support of a generous community of loved ones, friends and allies. I'm deeply grateful to everyone who helped me accomplish this goal.

Loving thanks to my amazing husband Jimm, for being a perfect sounding board, editor at all hours, unconditional cheering section, and for cooking dinner almost every night for a full year.

Lifetimes of gratitude go to Leonard A. Wisneski, MD, FACP, who encouraged the idea for this book at an unforgettable meeting in San Diego. Your vision and guidance have made all the difference.

Heartfelt appreciation goes to Midge Murphy, JD, PhD (Energy Medicine), for her caring, intuitive wisdom and invaluable support.

Grateful acknowledgment goes to Paul J. Mills, PhD, whose kind generosity and patience were instrumental in getting the research across the finish line.

Much love goes to Jeannette Bondurant of Larimar J Communications for savvy advice, meticulous research, and undaunted friendship.

Immense gratitude goes to the doctors, nurses, colleagues, and clients who generously contributed their inspirational personal stories. It is an honor to share them.

A mighty thank you goes to Fiona Robertson, Daniel Culver, Joanne Osborn, Glen Wilkins, and the team at Watkins Publishing for their enthusiasm in the subject and their gracious support. Grateful thanks to Bill Gladstone of Waterside Productions, who immediately understood the vision for this book and was willing to champion it.

I give heartfelt acknowledgment to the following wonderful souls, without whom this book would have never gotten past page one: intrepid coach and editor Kimberly Lord Stewart, whose great humor and positivity kept the engine running; Linda Negrin for peerless and cheerful efficiency; Melva Colter for excellent transcriptions and keen eye; Donna Agan, for organizing the data and helping me to understand it; and Teri Wilder and Sue Perisi for keeping me on track.

For their invaluable contributions, I wish to thank: Wil Alaura, AADP; Christine Allison, RN, BSN, CMIP; Sheryl Attig, PhD; Larry Burk, MD, CEHP; Lloyd Costello, MD, MA (Spiritual Psychology); Larry Dossey, MD; Frank Faltus, MD; Maria Gentile, DO, CMIP; Shamini Jain, PhD; Mary Louise Coan, MD, PhD; Gladys T. McGarey, MD, MD(H); Marie Mendoza-Cipollo, DC, CMIP, HC; Diane Puchbauer, PsyD; Cay Randall-May, PhD; Natasha Reiss, LAc, MSTOM, CMIP; Sandy Robertson, RN, MSN, HNB-BC, CHTP, CMIP; Winter Robinson, LCP; Holly Scalmanini, LAc; Karandeep Singh, MD; Lucia Thornton, ThD, MSN, RN, AHN-BC; Elizabeth Thorson, RN; Stephanie Valenzuela, CMIP; and Helané Wahbeh, ND, MCR.

I owe a huge debt of gratitude to the medical–scientific–spiritual visionaries who are paving the way for a more intuitive world of healthcare, and are engaged in building a strong community of like-minded spirits. To those who were willing to endorse a newcomer laser-focused on her mission, I am forever grateful for your support: Mimi Guarneri, MD, FACC, ABOIM, and Rauni Prittinen King, RN, MIH, BSN, CHTP/I, HNB-BC, at Pacific Pearl La Jolla; Tabatha Parker, ND, Erika Cappelluti, MD, PhD, MA, FCCP, ABOIM, and April Gruzinsky, MS, at the Academy of Integrative Health & Medicine; Chris Moline-Messick, RN, BSN, C, FAACVPR, Marcie Hintz, MBA, CJAT, HTPA, and Jacqueline Watson, RN, at CTC, Scripps Memorial Hospital; and Devorah Coryell, Director, Andrew Weil Center for Integrative Medicine IMER Program.

Warmest appreciation goes to Rev. Tiffany Barsotti, MTh, CHt, MCPLT, CCT; Lori Johnson, RN, MSN, OCN, AHN-BC; Sharon Wampler and John Newsam; Kathy Cueva and Bob Bowen at the Reiki Wind School & Healing Center, and many more in the San Diego energy healing community.

My parents helped me find my authentic voice and place in the world. I am grateful for my magnificent mother, Bruria Finkel, who filled our home with images of spiritual mysteries and whose intuitive artistic confidence imbued my life, and for my brilliant father, David Finkel, who taught me how to examine, inquire and reflect, and to stand up for what I believe.

A special thanks goes to my "magical aunts," Gilah Hirsch and Hella Hammid, who propped open the door to spiritual awareness and community. Deepest gratitude goes to all of my spiritual teachers who have shined a light on my path throughout the years.

This book is written for my incredible students who continually inspire me with their dedication to changing the paradigm of healthcare with medical intuition. The future is waiting for you.

ABOUT THE AUTHOR

Wendie Colter, MCWC, CMIP, is the founder and CEO of The Practical Path, Inc., presenting intuitive development for wellness professionals. The company name reflects her mission to fuse spiritual wisdom traditions with constructive, real-world results. A Certified Medical Intuitive Practitioner and Master Certified Wellness Coach, she has maintained a thriving private practice for more than 20 years and has been teaching intuitive development and energy healing professionally for 14 years. Wendie is an invited instructor and speaker at prominent health and education organizations and a regular guest on radio, summits and podcasts. Her trailblazing research on medical intuition is published in the *Journal of Alternative and Complementary Medicine* (*JACM*). Wendie serves on the Integrative Health Policy Consortium's (IHPC) BioEnergy & Health Committee, the Consciousness & Healing Initiative's CHI Healing Practitioners Council, and the working group of the National Organization for Professional Medical Intuition (NOPMI). Her accredited certification program in medical intuition, Medical Intuitive Training, has been pivotal in helping holistic health professionals from every discipline develop and optimize their inherent intuition. Wendie's commitment to the deeper awareness and understanding of the balance between body, mind and spirit is evident in her transformative programs, workshops and consultations.

For more information, please visit www.thepracticalpath.com

The Practical Path®, Inc.
Intuitive Development for Wellness Professionals®
- Medical Intuitive Training™ Practitioner Certification Program
- Medical Intuition for Healing Workshop™
- Guided Meditations Audio Series

ENDNOTES

Introduction
1   Patrick, G. Thomas White, & Chapman, F. Miller. (1935). *Introduction to Philosophy.* Houghton Mifflin. (p.44).

Chapter I
1   Inglis, B. (1989). *The Unknown Guest: The Mystery of Intuition.* Coronet/Hodder & Stoughton. (p.145).
2   Hermanns, W. (1983). *Einstein and the Poet: In Search of the Cosmic Man.* Branden Publishing Co. (p.103).
3   Peterkin, A. (2017). Physician Intuition. *Canadian Medical Association Journal, 189*(14), E544; Melin-Johansson, C., Palmqvist, R., and Rönnberg, L. (2017). Clinical Intuition in the Nursing Process and Decision-Making: A Mixed-Studies Review. *Journal of Clinical Nursing, 26*(23–24), 3936–3949; Marks-Tarlow, T. (2012). *Clinical Intuition in Psychotherapy: The Neurobiology of Embodied Response (Norton Series on Interpersonal Neurobiology)* (Illustrated ed.). W. W. Norton & Company; Van Hoesen, K., MD, Corbitt, A. D. (2018). *Medical Intuition: UCSD* [Video]. Retrieved September 26, 2021, from https://www.youtube.com/watch?v=fNbd5o_V0Lw&t=351s
4   Random House. *Intuition.* (2010). Random House Kernerman Webster's College Dictionary. Retrieved November 2, 2021, from https://www.dictionary.com/browse/intuition

5   Gannotta, R., Malik, S., Chan, A. Y., Urgun, K., Hsu, F., & Vadera, S. (2018). Integrative Medicine as a Vital Component of Patient Care. *Cureus, 3098.*

6   U.S. Department of Veterans Affairs, *Whole Health.* U.S. Department of Veterans Affairs. Retrieved June 12, 2021, from https://www.va.gov/wholehealth/

7   Dossey, L. (2014). *One Mind: How Our Individual Mind Is Part of a Greater Consciousness and Why it Matters.* Hay House Inc. (pp.xxvi, 189–194).

8   Leskowitz, E. (2001). Chapter 13: Medical Intuition. In S. Shannon (Ed.), *Handbook of Complementary and Alternative Therapies in Mental Health.* Academic Press. (p.275).

9   Jowett, B. (Translator) (2019). In *Charmides: or Temperance by Plato (written 380 B.C.E.).* Independently Published. (pp.154–160). Retrieved November 2, 2021, from http://classics.mit.edu/Plato/charmides.html

10 Eccles, J. C., & Popper, K. (1991). *Evolution of the Brain: Creation of the Self* (1st ed.). Routledge. (p.241).

11 Koenig, H. G., Hooten, E. G., Lindsay-Calkins, E., & Meador, K. G. (2010). Spirituality in Medical School Curricula: Findings from a National Survey. *The International Journal of Psychiatry in Medicine, 40*(4), 391–398.

12 Puchalski, C. M., Blatt, B., Kogan, M., Butler, A. (2014). Spirituality and Health: The Development of a Field. *Academic Medicine, 89*(1).

13 Bechtel, W, & Williamson, R. C. (1998). Vitalism. *Routledge Encyclopedia of Philosophy.* Routledge; Coulter, I., Snider, P., & Neil, A. (2019). Vitalism – A Worldview Revisited: A Critique of Vitalism and Its Implications for Integrative Medicine. *Integrative Medicine (Encinitas, Calif.), 18*(3), 60–73.

14 Kaptchuk, T. J., & Eisenberg, D. M. (1998). Chiropractic. *Archives of Internal Medicine, 158*(20), 2215–2224; Masiello, D. J. (1999). Osteopathy – A

Philosophical Perspective: Reflections on Sutherland's Experience of the Tide. *Journal of the American Academy of Osteopathy*, *9*(2), 22–39; Standish, L. J., Calabrese, C., & Snider, P. (2006). The Naturopathic Medical Research Agenda: The Future and Foundation of Naturopathic Medical Science. *The Journal of Alternative and Complementary Medicine*, *12*(3), 341–345.

15 Chrisman, L. (2005). *Energy Medicine. The Gale Encyclopedia of Alternative Medicine* (2nd ed.). Thompson Gale. (p. 687).

16 Rubik, B., Muehsam, D., Hammerschlag, R., & Jain, S. (2015). Biofield Science and Healing: History, Terminology, and Concepts. *Global Advances in Health and Medicine*, *4*(Suppl), 8–14.

17 Hammerschlag, R., Levin, M., McCraty, R., Bat, N., Ives, J. A., Lutgendorf, S. K., & Oschman, J. L. (2015). Biofield Physiology: A Framework for an Emerging Discipline. *Global Advances in Health and Medicine*, *4*(Suppl), 35–41; Jain. S. (2021). *Healing Ourselves: Biofield Science and the Future of Health*. Sounds True. (pp.160–168).

18 Hubacher, J. (2015). The Phantom Leaf Effect: A Replication, Part 1. *The Journal of Alternative and Complementary Medicine*, *21*(2), 83–90.

19 Shields, D., Fuller, A., Resnicoff, M., Butcher, H. K., & Frisch, N. (2016). Human Energy Field: A Concept Analysis. *Journal of Holistic Nursing*, *35*(4), 352–368; Dale, C. (2009). *The Subtle Body: An Encyclopedia of Your Energetic Anatomy* (Illustrated ed.). Sounds True. (pp.147–155, 251–268).

20 Shealy, C. N. (2010). *Medical Intuition: Awakening to Wholeness*. 4th Dimension Press. (p.106).

21 Colter, W. (June 12, 2021). *Measuring the Accuracy of Medical Intuition: A Groundbreaking Study*. [Presentation]. American Holistic Nurses Association (AHNA), 41st Annual Conference.

22 Weiss, T., & Swede, M. J. (2019). Transforming Preprofessional Health Education through Relationship-Centered Care and Narrative Medicine. *Teaching and Learning in Medicine, 31*(2), 222–233.

Chapter 2

1   Institute of Medicine, Committee on the Use of Complementary and Alternative Medicine by the American Public. (2005). *Complementary and Alternative Medicine in the United States: Appendix A, CAM Therapies, Practices and Systems.* National Academies Press.

2   Benor, D. (2001). *Intuitive Assessments: An Overview.* Copyright © Daniel J. Benor, M.D. 2001. Reprinted with permission of the author P.O. Box 76 Bellmawr, NJ 08099 www.WholisticHealingResearch.com DB@danielbenor.com

3   Murphy, M. (2020). *Practice Energy Healing in Integrity: The Joy of Offering Your Gifts Legally and Ethically.* Territorial Publishing. (pp.2, 8).

4   National Center for Complementary Integrative Health (2021). *Complementary, Alternative, or Integrative Health: What's In a Name?* National Institutes of Health. Retrieved July 19, 2021, from www.nccih.nih.gov/

5   Colter, W., & Mills, P. J. (2020). Assessing the Accuracy of Medical Intuition: A Subjective and Exploratory Study. *The Journal of Alternative and Complementary Medicine, 26*(12), 1130–1135. Mary Ann Liebert, Inc. publishers.

6   Colter, W. (June 12, 2021). *Measuring the Accuracy of Medical Intuition: A Groundbreaking Study.* [Presentation]. American Holistic Nurses Association (AHNA), 41st Annual Conference.

7   Carver, N., Gupta, V., & Hipskind, J. E. (2021). Medical Error. *StatPearls.* StatPearls Publishing. Retrieved November 2, 2021, from https://pubmed.ncbi.nlm.nih.gov/28613514/

8   Makary, M. A. (May 3, 2016). Medical Error – The
     Third Leading Cause of Death in the US. *The BMJ, 353*;
     Daniel, M. (May 3, 2016). *Study Suggests Medical Errors
     Now Third Leading Cause of Death in the U.S.* Johns
     Hopkins Medicine, News and Publications. Retrieved
     November 2, 2021, from https://www.hopkinsmedicine.
     org/news/media/releases/study_suggests_medical_errors_
     now_third_leading_cause_of_death_in_the_us Note:
     COVID-19 replaced medical error as the third leading
     cause of death in 2020.

9   James, J. T. (2013). A New, Evidence-Based Estimate of
     Patient Harms Associated with Hospital Care. *Journal of
     Patient Safety, 9*(3), 122–128.

10   Graber, M. L. (2013). The Incidence of Diagnostic Error
     in Medicine. *BMJ Quality & Safety, 22*(Suppl 2), ii21–
     ii27.

11   ECRI. (n.d.). *Diagnostic Errors, Maternal Health
     Top ECRI's 2020 Patient Safety Concerns.* ECRI.
     Retrieved October 24, 2021, from www.ecri.org/
     press/diagnostic-errors-maternal-health-top-ecri-2020-
     patient-safety-concerns/; Carbajal, E., Masson, G., &
     Bean, M. (December 30, 2020). *10 Top Patient Safety
     Issues for 2021.* Becker's Hospital Review. Retrieved
     October 24, 2021, from www.beckershospitalreview.com/
     patient-safety-outcomes/10-top-patient-safety-issues-
     for-2021.html

12   Washington Health Alliance. (February, 2018). *First, Do
     No Harm.* Washington Health Alliance. (p.6). Retrieved
     October 24, 2021, from www.wacommunitycheckup.org/
     media/47156/2018-first-do-no-harm.pdf; Kaiser Health
     News. (2017). *Unnecessary Medical Tests, Treatments Cost
     $200 Billion Annually, Cause Harm.* Healthcare Finance
     News. Retrieved March 4, 2021, from https://www.
     healthcarefinancenews.com/news/unnecessary-medical-
     tests-treatments-cost-200-billion-annually-cause-harm

13 Lyu, H., Xu, T., Brotman, D., Mayer-Blackwell, B., Cooper, M., Daniel, M., Wick, E. C., Saini, V., Brownlee, S., & Makary, M. A. (2017). Overtreatment in the United States. *PLoS ONE, 12*(9), e0181970.

14 Royce, C. S., Hayes, M. M., & Schwartzstein, R. M. (2019). Teaching Critical Thinking: A Case for Instruction in Cognitive Biases to Reduce Diagnostic Errors and Improve Patient Safety. *Academic Medicine: Journal of the Association of American Medical Colleges, 94*(2), 187–194.

15 Saposnik, G., Redelmeier, D., Ruff, C. C., & Tobler, P. N. (2016). Cognitive Biases Associated with Medical Decisions: A Systematic Review. *BMC Medical Informatics and Decision Making, 16*(1), 138; Becker's Healthcare. (June 9, 2017). *Becker's Hospital Review: How 4 Types of Cognitive Bias Contribute to Physician Diagnostic Errors – and How to Overcome Them.* Becker's Healthcare. Retrieved October 24, 2021, from www.beckershospitalreview.com/hospital-physician-relationships/how-4-types-of-cognitive-bias-contribute-to-physician-diagnostic-errors-and-how-to-overcome-it. html

16 Berman, A. C., & Chutka, D. S. (2016). Assessing Effective Physician–Patient Communication Skills: "Are You Listening to Me, Doc?" *Korean Journal of Medical Education, 28*(2), 243–249; Martin, L. R., Williams, S. L., Haskard, K. B., & Dimatteo, M. R. (2005). The Challenge of Patient Adherence. *Therapeutics and Clinical Risk Management, 1*(3), 189–199.

17 Reith, T. P. (2018). Burnout in United States Healthcare Professionals: A Narrative Review. *Cureus, 10*(12), e3681; Boyle, D. A. (2015). Compassion Fatigue. *Nursing, 45*(7), 48–51; Kalmoe, M. C., Chapman, M. B., Gold, J. A., & Giedinghagen, A. M. (2019). Physician Suicide: A Call to Action. *Missouri Medicine, 116*(3), 211–216.

18   Murphy, M. (2020). *Practice Energy Healing in Integrity: The Joy of Offering Your Gifts Legally and Ethically.* Territorial Publishing.

19   Cohen, M. H. (2002). *Future Medicine: Ethical Dilemmas, Regulatory Challenges, and Therapeutic Pathways to Health Care and Healing in Human Transformation.* University of Michigan Press.

Chapter 3

1   Gauld, A. (1992). *A History of Hypnotism.* Cambridge University Press. (pp.1–4).

2   Ibid. (pp.39–52).

3   Inglis, B. (1977). *Natural and Supernatural: A History of the Paranormal from the Earliest Times to 1914.* White Crow Books. (p.135).

4   Deleuze, J. P. F., & Hartshorn, T. C. (2019). *Practical Instruction in Animal Magnetism* (Triamazikamno Editions). Independently published. (p.157).

5   Inglis, B. (1977). *Natural and Supernatural: A History of the Paranormal from the Earliest Times to 1914.* White Crow Books. (p.140).

6   Gauld, A. (1992). *A History of Hypnotism.* Cambridge University Press. (pp.53–57).

7   Inglis, B. (1977). *Natural and Supernatural: A History of the Paranormal from the Earliest Times to 1914.* White Crow Books. (p.144).

8   Ibid. (pp.139–140).

9   Gauld, A. (1992). A History of Hypnotism. Cambridge University Press. (pp.26–27); Inglis, B. (1977). *Natural and Supernatural: A History of the Paranormal from the Earliest Times to 1914.* White Crow Books. (pp.133–4).

10   Gauld, A. (1992). *A History of Hypnotism.* Cambridge University Press. (pp.26, 133–134); Inglis, B. (1977). *Natural and Supernatural: A History of the Paranormal*

from the Earliest Times to 1914. White Crow Books. (pp.147–150).

11 Inglis, B. (1977). *Natural and Supernatural: A History of the Paranormal from the Earliest Times to 1914.* White Crow Books. (p.149).

12 Ibid. (pp.157–158).

13 Robertson, D. (2019). *Beginners Guide to the History of Hypnosis (Timeline).* The UK College of Hypnosis and Hypnotherapy – Hypnotherapy Training Courses. Retrieved May 20, 2021, from www.ukhypnosis.com

14 Haller, J. S. (2010). *Swedenborg, Mesmer, and the Mind/ Body Connection: The Roots of Complementary Medicine (Swedenborg Studies)* (1st ed.). Swedenborg Foundation Publishers. (pp.138–145).

15 Apkarian-Russell, P. E. (2006). *Washington's Haunted Past: Capital Ghosts of America (Haunted America)* (Illustrated ed.). The History Press. (pp.44–45).

16 Haller, J. S. (2010). *Swedenborg, Mesmer, and the Mind/ Body Connection: The Roots of Complementary Medicine (Swedenborg Studies)* (1st ed.). Swedenborg Foundation Publishers. (p.131).

17 Carmack, S. D. (2020). *In Search of Maria B. Hayden: The American Medium Who Brought Spiritualism to the U.K.* Scattered Leaves Press. (pp.227, 229–231); Inglis, B. (2012). *Natural and Supernatural: A History of the Paranormal from the Earliest Times to 1914.* White Crow Books. (pp.205–210).

18 Mayr, E. (2010). The Decline of Vitalism. In M. A. Bedau & C. E. Cleland (Eds.), *The Nature of Life: Classical and Contemporary Perspectives from Philosophy and Science.* Cambridge University Press. (pp.93–95).

19 Quimby, P. P., & Seale, E. (1988). *The Complete Writings: Vol 3* (1st ed.). DeVorss & Co.; Hughes, R. (2002). *An Extract from a Letter, December 1859.* Phineas Parkhurst Quimby Resource Center. Retrieved October 25, 2021,

from www.ppquimby.com/articles/extract_from_a_letter_an.htm

20 Haller, J. S. (2010). *Swedenborg, Mesmer, and the Mind/Body Connection: The Roots of Complementary Medicine (Swedenborg Studies)* (1st ed.). Swedenborg Foundation Publishers. (pp.159–166).

21 Dresser, H. W. (2021). *A History of the New Thought Movement* (Illustrated ed.). Independently published. (pp.12–13).

22 Hughes, R. (2002). *Home Page.* Phineas Parkhurst Quimby Resource Center. Retrieved October 25, 2021, from https://www.ppquimby.com/index.html

23 McGarey, W. A. (1997). *The Edgar Cayce Remedies.* Bantam Doubleday Dell Publishing Group. (p.16).

24 Sugrue, T. (1999). *There Is a River: The Story of Edgar Cayce* (50th Anniversary ed.). A.R.E. Press.

25 Smith, R. A. (Ed.) (2021). *History of the Edgar Cayce Hospital.* Venture Inward Magazine. Edgar Cayce's A.R.E. Retrieved July 19, 2021, from www.edgarcayce.org

26 Sugrue, T. (1999). *There Is a River: The Story of Edgar Cayce* (50th Anniversary ed.). A.R.E. Press. (pp.290–291).

27 Shreiner, A. B., Kao, J. Y., & Young, V. B. (2015). The Gut Microbiome in Health and in Disease. *Current Opinion in Gastroenterology, 31*(1), 69–75; Bland J. (2016). The Gut Mucosal Firewall and Functional Medicine. *Integrative Medicine (Encinitas, Calif.), 15*(4), 19–22.

28 Edgar Cayce's A.R.E. (2021). *Holistic Health Database: Therapies.* Edgar Cayce's A.R.E. Retrieved July 20, 2021, from www.edgarcayce.org

29 Myss, C. (1996). *Anatomy of the Spirit: The Seven Stages of Power and Healing* (1st ed.). Harmony. (p.58).

30 Myss, C. (1996). *Anatomy of the Spirit: The Seven Stages of Power and Healing* (1st ed.). Harmony.

31 Winfrey, O. (December 10, 2012). *Caroline Myss Interview with Oprah Winfrey.* Oprah.com. Retrieved July 20, 2021, from www.oprah.com

32 Myss, C., & Shealy, C. N. (1993). *The Creation of Health: The Emotional, Psychological, and Spiritual Responses that Promote Health and Healing* (Three Rivers Press ed.). Harmony. (p.72).

33 Shealy, C. N. (2010). *Medical Intuition: Your Awakening to Wholeness* (Illustrated ed.). 4th Dimension Press. (p.12).

34 Lowes, R. (September 17, 2004). *A Field Guide to Alternative Healers.* Medical Economics, *81*(21); Sorgen, C. (January 3, 2003). *Intuition and Medicine: More Than a Feeling.* WebMD. Retrieved October 3, 2021, from https://www.webmd.com/balance/features/more-than-feeling; Zablocki, E. (April, 2020). Medical Intuition – Using the Sixth Sense in Integrative Health Practice. *Townsend Letter, 441*, pp.14–15; Stewart, K. (January 7, 2021). New Study Shows High Accuracy of Medical Intuition. *Today's Practitioner.* Retrieved October 3, 2021, from https://todayspractitioner.com/mind-body-medicine/new-study-shows-high-accuracy-of-medical-intuition/#.YVpnaEJKjGY; Martin, K. (December 24, 2019). *We All Have Medical Intuition – Now Here's How to Use It.* Goop. Retrieved July 22, 2021, from www.goop.com; Russell, J. (July, 1998). The "Doctors" Who Feel Your Pain. *Good Housekeeping,* pp.106–109, 166–167.

35 OWN. (February 5, 2011). *Medical Intuition, Miracle Detectives. The Oprah Winfrey Network.* [Video]. YouTube. Retrieved October 3, 2021, from https://www.youtube.com/watch?v=SjCOiOeZS8U; The Doctors. (July 14, 2016). *Medical Intuitive?* The Doctors. [Video]. YouTube. Retrieved October 3, 2021, from https://www.youtube.com/watch?v=C7bwY0ASfk4; John Kortum and Dr Oz. (February 2, 2014). *Medical Intuitive John Kortum and Dr. Oz Exploring Life Span Moisture Levels.* Dr. Oz.

[Video]. YouTube. Retrieved October 3, 2021, from
https://www.youtube.com/watch?v=kiyg_uskKLc&t=53s

36 Orloff, J. (2010). *Second Sight: An Intuitive Psychiatrist Tells Her Extraordinary Story and Shows You How to Tap Your Own Inner Wisdom* (Reissue ed.). Harmony; Schulz, M. L. N. (1998). *Awakening Intuition: Using Your Mind-Body Network for Insight and Healing* (2nd Printing ed.). Harmony Books.

Chapter 4

1 Radin, D. I., & Schlitz, M. J. (2005). Gut Feelings, Intuition, and Emotions: An Exploratory Study. *The Journal of Alternative and Complementary Medicine, 11*(1), 85–91; McCraty, R., Atkinson, M., & Bradley, R. T. (2004). Electrophysiological Evidence of Intuition: Part 2. A System-Wide Process? *The Journal of Alternative and Complementary Medicine, 10*(2), 325–336; Pretz, J. E., Brookings, J. B., Carlson, L. A., Humbert, T. K., Roy, M., Jones, M., & Memmert, D. (2014). Development and Validation of a New Measure of Intuition: The Types of Intuition Scale. *Journal of Behavioral Decision Making, 27*(5), 454–467; Dörfler, V., & Ackermann, F. (2012). Understanding Intuition: The Case for Two Forms of Intuition. *Management Learning, 43*(5), 545–564.

2 Roseman-Halsband, J. L., Marcow Speiser, V., & Lafferty, L. (2017). Intuition in Medicine. *Alternative and Complementary Therapies, 23*(6), 231–235; Van den Brink, N., Holbrechts, B., Brand, P. L. P., Stolper, E. C. F., & van Royen, P. (2019). Role of Intuitive Knowledge in the Diagnostic Reasoning of Hospital Specialists: A Focus Group Study. *BMJ Open, 9*(1), e022724.

3 Greenhalgh, T. (2002). Intuition and Evidence – Uneasy Bedfellows? *The British Journal of General Practice: The Journal of the Royal College of General Practitioners, 52*(478), 395–400.

4   Mickleborough, T. (2015). Intuition in Medical Practice: A Reflection on Donald Schön's Reflective Practitioner. *Medical Teacher*, *37*(10), 889–891.

5   Woolley, A., & Kostopoulou, O. (2013). Clinical Intuition in Family Medicine: More Than First Impressions. *The Annals of Family Medicine*, *11*(1), 60–66.

6   Ibid.

7   Billay, D., Myrick, F., Luhanga, F., & Yonge, O. (2007). A Pragmatic View of Intuitive Knowledge in Nursing Practice. *Nursing Forum*, *42*(3), 147–155; Rew, L. (1986). Intuition: Concept Analysis of a Group Phenomenon. *Advances in Nursing Science*, *8*(2), 21–28; Hassani, P. (2016). State of Science, "Intuition in Nursing Practice": A Systematic Review Study. *Journal of Clinical and Diagnostic Research*, *10*(2), JE07–JE11; Nibbelink, C. W., & Brewer, B. B. (2018). Decision-Making in Nursing Practice: An Integrative Literature Review. *Journal of Clinical Nursing*, *27*(5–6), 917–928.

8   Dossey, B. M., & Keegan, L. (2009). *Holistic Nursing – A Handbook for Practice* (5th ed.). Jones & Bartlet. (p.147).

9   Melin-Johansson, C., Palmqvist, R., & Rönnberg, L. (2017). Clinical Intuition in the Nursing Process and Decision-Making – a Mixed-Studies Review. *Journal of Clinical Nursing*, *26*(23–24), 3936–3949.

10 Brush, J. E., Sherbino, J., & Norman, G. R. (2017). How Expert Clinicians Intuitively Recognize a Medical Diagnosis. *The American Journal of Medicine*, *130*(6), 629–634; Vanstone, M., Monteiro, S., Colvin, E., Norman, G., Sherbino, J., Sibbald, M., Dore, K., & Peters, A. (2019). Experienced Physician Descriptions of Intuition in Clinical Reasoning: A Typology. *Diagnosis*, *6*(3), 259–268; Polge, J. (1995). Critical Thinking: The Use of Intuition in Making Clinical Nursing Judgments. *The Journal of the New York State Nurses' Association*, *26*(2), 4–9.

11   Liem, T. (2017). Intuitive Judgement in the Context
of Osteopathic Clinical Reasoning. *The Journal of the
American Osteopathic Association, 117*(9), 586–594.

12   Miller, E. M., Hill, P. D. (2018). Intuition in Clinical
Decision Making: Differences Among Practicing Nurses.
Journal of Holistic Nursing, 36(4), 318–329.

13   Rew, L., & Barrow, E. M., Jr. (2007). State of the
Science: Intuition in Nursing, A Generation of Studying
the Phenomenon. *Advances in Nursing Science, 30*(1),
E15–E25.

14   Marks-Tarlow, T. (2012). *Clinical Intuition in
Psychotherapy: The Neurobiology of Embodied Response
(Norton Series on Interpersonal Neurobiology)* (Illustrated
ed.). W. W. Norton & Company. (pp.3, 30, 32, 42, 163,
188); Sinclair, M. (2005). Intuition: Myth or a Decision-
Making Tool? *Management Learning, 36*(3), 353–370.

15   Benor, D. (2001). *Intuitive Assessments: An Overview.*
Copyright © Daniel J. Benor, M.D. 2001. Reprinted
with permission of the author P.O. Box 76 Bellmawr,
NJ 08099 www.WholisticHealingResearch.com DB@
danielbenor.com

16   Colter, W. (2021). *Medical Intuitive Training™*. The
Practical Path®, Inc. Retrieved July 26, 2021, from
https://thepracticalpath.com

17   Colter, W., & Mills, P. J. (2020). Assessing the Accuracy
of Medical Intuition: A Subjective and Exploratory Study.
*The Journal of Alternative and Complementary Medicine,
26*(12), 1130–1135. Mary Ann Liebert, Inc. publishers.

18   Attig, S., & Schwartz, G. (April 2006). *Remote
Diagnosis of Medical Conditions: A Double-Blind
Experiment of Medical Intuition.* Presented at the
seventh biennial interdisciplinary conference, The
Science of Consciousness, organized by the Center for
Consciousness Studies. Dept. of Psychology, University of
Arizona, Tucson, AZ; Interview with study author Sheryl
Attig, PhD, May 1, 2020.

19 Ibid.
20 Cayce, E. E., & Cayce, H. L. (1971). *The Outer Limits of Edgar Cayce's Power.* Harper & Row. (pp.14, 21–24).
21 Karagulla, S. (1967). *Breakthrough to Creativity: Your Higher Sense Perception.* DeVorss & Co. (pp.123–146, 254–261).
22 Shealy, C. N. (2010). *Medical Intuition: Your Awakening to Wholeness.* A.R.E. Press/4th Dimension Press. (p.135–136).
23 Ibid.; Shealy, C. N. (1976). Perspectives on Psychic Diagnosis. *The A.R.E. Journal, 11*(5), 208–217.
24 Myss, C., & Shealy, C. N. (1993). *The Creation of Health: The Emotional, Psychological, and Spiritual Responses that Promote Health and Healing* (Three Rivers Press ed.). Harmony. (p.72).
25 Ibid. (p.59).
26 Ibid. (pp.65–66).
27 Young, D. E., & Aung, S. K. H. (1997). An Experimental Test of Psychic Diagnosis of Disease. *The Journal of Alternative and Complementary Medicine, 3*(1), 39–53.
28 Ibid.
29 Jobst, K. A. (1997). One Man's Meat Is Another Man's Poison: The Challenge of Psychic/Intuitive Diagnosis to the Diagnostic Paradigm of Orthodox Medical Science. *The Journal of Alternative and Complementary Medicine, 3*(1), 1–3.
30 Burk, L., O'Brien, B., Charron, J. M., Sherman, K. J., & Bullock, M. L. (1997). Psychic/Intuitive Diagnosis: Two Case Reports and Commentary. *The Journal of Alternative and Complementary Medicine, 3*(3), 209–211.
31 Burk, L. (2012). *Let Magic Happen: Adventures in Healing with a Holistic Radiologist.* Healing Imager Press. (p.59–61).
32 Benor, D. (2001). *Intuitive Assessments: An Overview.* Copyright © Daniel J. Benor, M.D. 2001. Reprinted with permission of the author P.O. Box 76 Bellmawr,

NJ 08099 www.WholisticHealingResearch.com DB@ danielbenor.com

33 Benor, D. (1992). Intuitive Diagnosis. *Subtle Energies & Energy Medicine Journal, 3*(2), 4–64.

34 Amoils, S. (2002). The Diagnostic Validity of Human Electromagnetic Field (Aura) Perception. *Medical Acupuncture, 13*(2), 25–28.

35 Ibid. (p.25).

36 Ibid. (p.28).

37 Vaughan, A. (1974). Investigation of Silva Mind Control Claims. In W. G. Roll, R. L. Morris, & J. D. Morris (Eds.), *Research in Parapsychology 1973* (p.51). Scarecrow; Brier, R., Savitis, B., and Schmeidler, G. (1974). Experimental Tests of Silva Mind Control Graduates. In W. G. Roll, R. L. Morris, & J. D. Morris (Eds.), *Research in Parapsychology 1973* (pp.13–15). Scarecrow; Jacobson, N., & Wiklund, N. (1975). Investigation of Claims of Diagnosing by Means of ESP. In W. G. Roll, R. L. Morris, & J. D. Morris (Eds.), *Research in Parapsychology 1975* (pp.74–76). Scarecrow; Eisenberg, D. M., Davis, R. B., Waletzky, J., Yager, A., Landsberg, L., Aronson, M., Seibel, M., & Delbanco, T. L. (2000). Inability of an "Energy Transfer Diagnostician" to Distinguish between Fertile and Infertile Women. *MedGenMed: Medscape General Medicine, 3*(1).

Chapter 5

1 Colter, W. (June 12, 2021). *Measuring the Accuracy of Medical Intuition: A Groundbreaking Study.* [Presentation]. American Holistic Nurses Association (AHNA), 41st Annual Conference.

2 Johnson, P. K. (1998). *Edgar Cayce in Context: The Readings: Truth and Fiction (Suny Series in Western Esoteric*

Traditions). State University of New York Press. (pp.16, 17, 20, 25).

3   Ketchum, W. H. (1964). *The Discovery of Edgar Cayce* (1st ed.). A.R.E. Press.

4   Curry, L. E. (2008). *The Doctor and the Psychic.* BookSurge Publishing. (pp.44–45).

5   Myss, C., & Shealy, C. N. (1993). *The Creation of Health: The Emotional, Psychological, and Spiritual Responses that Promote Health and Healing.* (Three Rivers Press ed.). Harmony; Myss, C. (1996). *Anatomy of the Spirit:* Myss, C. (1996). *Anatomy of the Spirit: The Seven Stages of Power and Healing* (1st ed.). Harmony.

6   Wisneski, L. A. (2017). *The Scientific Basis of Integrative Health* (3rd ed.). CRC Press, Taylor & Francis Group. (p.245).

7   Mason, R. (2000). Expanding Diagnostic Vision with Medical Intuition. *Alternative and Complementary Therapies, 6*(6), 331–336.

8   Dean, S. R., Plyler, C. O. J., & Dean, M. L. (1980). Should Psychic Studies Be Included in Psychiatric Education? An Opinion Survey. *American Journal of Psychiatry, 137*(10), 1247–1249.

9   Srivastava, A., & Grube, M. (2009). Does Intuition Have a Role in Psychiatric Diagnosis? *Psychiatric Quarterly, 80*(2), 99–106.

10 Zhao, J., & Xu, J. J. (2018). Experimental Study on Application of Polypropylene Hernia of Fat Stem Cells in Rats. *European Review for Medical and Pharmacological Sciences, 22*(18), 6156–6161.

11 Randall-May, C. (2014). *Inner Visions of Matter and Subtle Energy.* CayMay Press.

Chapter 6

1   American Psychological Association. (2020). *Spontaneous Remission.* APA Dictionary of Psychology. Retrieved July

26, 2021, from https://dictionary.apa.org/spontaneous-remission; Institute of Noetic Sciences (IONS). (2021). *Spontaneous Remission Bibliography*. IONS. Retrieved July 26, 2021, from https://noetic.org/science/spontaneous-remission-bibliography/

2   National Center for Complementary and Integrative Health. (February 10, 2015). *Nationwide Survey Reveals Widespread Use of Mind and Body Practices*. [Press release]. National Center for Complementary and Integrative Health. Retrieved February 17, 2021, from https://www.nccih.nih.gov/news/press-releases/nationwide-survey-reveals-widespread-use-of-mind-and-body-practices

3   Jonas, W. B., & Rosenbaum, E. (2021). The Case for Whole-Person Integrative Care. *Medicina, 57*(7), 677.

4   U.S. Department of Veterans Affairs, *Whole Health*. U.S. Department of Veterans Affairs. Retrieved July 26, 2021, from www.va.gov/wholehealth/

5   Champion, L., Economides, M., & Chandler, C. (2018). The Efficacy of a Brief App-Based Mindfulness Intervention on Psychosocial Outcomes in Healthy Adults: A Pilot Randomised Controlled Trial. *PLoS ONE, 13*(12), e0209482.

6   The Free Dictionary. (2009). *Mind-Body Medicine*. TheFreeDictionary.com. Retrieved April 30, 2021, from https://medical-dictionary.thefreedictionary.com/mind-body+medicine

7   Random House. (2017). *The Random House Dictionary*. Random House, Inc.

8   Simonton, O. C., Matthews-Simonton, S., & Creighton, J. (1978). *Getting Well Again: A Step-By-Step Self-Help Guide to Overcoming Cancer for Patients and Their Families* (Bantam Reissue 1992 ed.). J P Tarcher, Inc. (pp.11, 88).

9   Nelson, V. J. (September 29, 2014). O. Carl Simonton Dies at 66; Oncologist Pioneered Mind-Body Connection to Fight Cancer. *Los Angeles Times*. www.latimes.com

10 Simonton, O. C. (1982). *CA: A Cancer Journal for Clinicians: Unproven Methods of Cancer Management, 32*(1), 58–61.

11 Niazi, A. K., & Niazi, S. K. (2011). Mindfulness-Based Stress Reduction: A Non-Pharmacological Approach for Chronic Illnesses. *North American Journal of Medical Sciences, 3*(1), 20–23.

12 Yeh, B. I., & Kong, I. D. (2013). The Advent of Lifestyle Medicine. *Journal of Lifestyle Medicine, 3*(1), 1–8; Clarke, C. A., & Hauser, M. E. (2016). Lifestyle Medicine: A Primary Care Perspective. *Journal of Graduate Medical Education, 8*(5), 665–667.

13 American Medical Association. (2012). *2012 Annual Meeting of the House of Delegates: Resolutions* (Issue Policy H-425.972). American Medical Association.

14 Simon & Schuster. (2021). *Deepak Chopra*. Simon & Schuster. Retrieved February 19, 2021, from www.simonandschuster.com/authors/Deepak-Chopra/1155961

15 Chopra, D. (2015). *Quantum Healing: Exploring the Frontiers of Mind/Body Medicine* (Revised, Updated ed.). Bantam. (p.300).

16 Chopra, D. (June 13, 2013). *7 Secrets to Grow Younger, Live Longer*. Chopra. Retrieved February 19, 2021, from https://chopra.com/articles/7-secrets-to-grow-younger-live-longer

17 Ballard, E. (April 20, 2012). Class Notes and Epiphanies from Oprah's Life Class with Deepak Chopra. *Psychology Today*. Retrieved November 4, 2021, from www.psychologytoday.com/gb/blog/epiphany/201204/class-notes-and-epiphanies-oprahs-lifeclass-deepak-chopra

18 Hay, L. (April 9, 2021). *About Louise Hay: Bio and Timeline of Achievements*. Louise Hay. Retrieved October 29, 2021, from www.louisehay.com/about/; Hay, L. (1984). *Heal Your Body* (4th ed.). Hay House Inc.; Hay, L. (1984). *You Can Heal Your Life* (Illustrated ed.). Hay House Inc.

19 A–Z Quotes. (December 7, 2010). *Top 25 Quotes by Louise Hay (of 471)*. [Facebook Post]. A–Z Quotes. Retrieved February 19, 2021, from www.azquotes.com/author/19603-Louise_Hay

20 Office of the Commissioner. (January, 1998). *Drug Study Designs. Guidance for Institutional Review Boards and Clinical Investigators*. U.S. Food and Drug Administration.

21 Patel, S. M., Stason, W. B., Legedza, A., Ock, S. M., Kaptchuk, T. J., Conboy, L., Canenguez, K., Park, J. K., Kelly, E., Jacobson, E., Kerr, C. E., & Lembo, A. J. (2005). The Placebo Effect in Irritable Bowel Syndrome Trials: A Meta-Analysis. *Neurogastroenterology and Motility: The Official Journal of the European Gastrointestinal Motility Society*, *17*(3), 332–340.

22 Zuckerman, A. (May 27, 2020). *46 Placebo Effect Statistics: 2020/2021 Data, Examples & Implications*. CompareCamp. Retrieved February 20, 2021, from https://comparecamp.com/placebo-effect-statistics

23 Brynie, F. (2009). *Brain Sense*. Amacom, HarperCollins Leadership. (pp.2, 24–25).

24 Jacobs, K. W., & Nordan, F. M. (1979). Classification of Placebo Drugs: Effect of Color. *Perceptual and Motor Skills*, *49*(2), 367–372.

25 Harvard Health Publishing. (April, 2012). *Putting the Placebo Effect to Work*. Harvard Health. Retrieved March 1, 2021, from www.health.harvard.edu/mind-and-mood/putting-the-placebo-effect-to-work

26 Schaefer, M., Sahin, T., & Berstecher, B. (2018). Why Do Open-Label Placebos Work? A Randomized Controlled Trial of an Open-Label Placebo Induction with and without Extended Information about the Placebo Effect in Allergic Rhinitis. *PLoS ONE*, *13*(3), e0192758.

27 Harvard Health Publishing. (May, 2017). *The Power of the Placebo Effect*. Harvard Health. Retrieved March 1, 2021,

from www.health.harvard.edu/mental-health/the-power-of-the-placebo-effect

28 Fässler, M., Meissner, K., Schneider, A., & Linde, K. (2010). Frequency and Circumstances of Placebo Use in Clinical Practice – A Systematic Review of Empirical Studies. *BMC Medicine, 8*(1).

29 Govender, S. (2015). *Is the Nocebo Effect Hurting Your Health?* WebMD. Retrieved March 21, 2021, from www.webmd.com/balance/features/is-the-nocebo-effect-hurting-your-health

30 Zuckerman, A. (May 27, 2020). *46 Placebo Effect Statistics: 2020/2021 Data, Examples & Implications.* CompareCamp. Retrieved February 20, 2021, from https://comparecamp.com/placebo-effect-statistics

31 Kosslyn, S., & Miller, W. G. (2015). *Top Brain, Bottom Brain: Harnessing the Power of the Four Cognitive Modes* (Revised ed.). Simon & Schuster.

32 Zhang, L., Qiu, F., Zhu, H., Xiang, M., & Zhou, L. (2019). Neural Efficiency and Acquired Motor Skills: An fMRI Study of Expert Athletes. *Frontiers in Psychology, 10*(2752).

33 Clark, T., & Williamon, A. (2011). Evaluation of a Mental Skills Training Program for Musicians. *Journal of Applied Sport Psychology, 23*(3), 342–359.

34 Krau, S. D. (2020). The Multiple Uses of Guided Imagery. *Nursing Clinics of North America, 55*(4), 467–474.

Chapter 7

1 Leonard, J. (June 3, 2020). *What is Trauma? What to Know.* Medical News Today. Retrieved November 10, 2021, from www.medicalnewstoday.com/articles/trauma

2 Braga, L. L., Mello, M. F., & Fiks, J. P. (2012). Transgenerational Transmission of Trauma and Resilience: A Qualitative Study with Brazilian Offspring of Holocaust Survivors. *BMC Psychiatry, 12*(1), 134.

3   Mayo Clinic. (July 6, 2018). *Post-traumatic Stress Disorder (PTSD) – Symptoms and Causes*. Mayo Clinic. Retrieved November 10, 2021, from www.mayoclinic.org/diseases-conditions/post-traumatic-stress-disorder/symptoms-causes/syc-20355967

4   Hannibal, S. (2003). The Hidden Language of Intuition. *The International Journal of Healing and Caring, 3*(1); Myss, C., & Shealy, C. N. (1993). *The Creation of Health: The Emotional, Psychological, and Spiritual Responses that Promote Health and Healing* (Three Rivers Press ed.). Harmony. (p.105); Myss, C. (1996). *Anatomy of the Spirit: The Seven Stages of Power and Healing* (1st ed.). Harmony. (p.xviii); Schulz, M. L. (1999). *Awakening Intuition: Using Your Mind-Body Network for Insight and Healing* (Illustrated ed.). Harmony. (pp.96–105).

5   van der Kolk, B. (2015). *The Body Keeps the Score: Brain, Mind, and Body in the Healing of Trauma*. Penguin. (p.21).

6   Felitti, V. J., Anda, R. F., Nordenberg, D., Williamson, D. F., Spitz, A. M., Edwards, V., Koss, M. P., & Marks, J. S. (2019). Relationship of Childhood Abuse and Household Dysfunction to Many of the Leading Causes of Death in Adults: The Adverse Childhood Experiences (ACE) Study. *American Journal of Preventive Medicine, 56*(6), 774–786.

7   Hughes, K., Bellis, M. A., Hardcastle, K. A., Sethi, D., Butchart, A., Mikton, C., Jones, L., & Dunne, M. P. (2017). The Effect of Multiple Adverse Childhood Experiences on Health: A Systematic Review and Meta-analysis. *The Lancet. Public Health, 2*(8), e356–e366.

8   Centers for Disease Control and Prevention. (2021). *CDC – BRFSS. Behavioral Risk Factor Surveillance System*. Centers for Disease Control and Prevention. Retrieved November 10, 2021, from www.cdc.gov/brfss/about/index.htm

9   Monnat, S. M., & Chandler, R. F. (2015). Long-Term

Physical Health Consequences of Adverse Childhood Experiences. *The Sociological Quarterly*, *56*(4), 723–752.

10   Centers for Disease Control and Prevention. (2020). *Preventing Adverse Childhood Experiences*. Centers for Disease Control and Prevention. Retrieved November 10, 2021, from www.cdc.gov/violenceprevention/aces/fastfact.html

11   Merrick, M. T., Ford, D. C., Ports, K. A., & Guinn, A. S. (2018). Prevalence of Adverse Childhood Experiences. From the 2011–2014 Behavioral Risk Factor Surveillance System in 23 States. *JAMA pediatrics*, *172*(11), 1038–1044.

12   Miller, T. R., Waehrer, G. M., Oh, D. L., Purewal Boparai, S., Ohlsson Walker, S., Silverio Marques, S., & Burke Harris, N. (2020). Adult Health Burden and Costs in California During 2013 Associated with Prior Adverse Childhood Experiences. *PLoS ONE*, *15*(1), e0228019.

13   Rank, O. (1929). *The Trauma of Birth*. Courier Corporation.

14   Entringer, S., Buss, C., & Wadhwa, P. D. (2015). Prenatal Stress, Development, Health and Disease Risk: A Psychobiological Perspective. Curt Richter Award Paper. *Psychoneuroendocrinology*, *62*, 366–375.

15   Chamberlain, D. B. (2013). *Windows to the Womb*. North Atlantic Books; Chamberlain, D. B. (1999). The Significance of Birth Memories. *Journal of Prenatal and Perinatal Psychology and Health*, *14*(1 and 2), 65–83.

16   Kiecolt-Glaser, J. K. (2009). Psychoneuroimmunology: Psychology's Gateway to the Biomedical Future. *Perspectives on Psychological Science*, *4*(4), 367–369.

17   Glaser, R., & Kiecolt-Glaser, J. K. (2005). Stress-Induced Immune Dysfunction: Implications for Health. *Nature Reviews Immunology*, *5*(3), 243–251.

18   Mathews, H. L., & Janusek, L. W. (2011). Epigenetics and Psychoneuroimmunology: Mechanisms and Models. *Brain, Behavior, and Immunity*, *25*(1), 25–39.

19 Dekel, R., & Goldblatt, H. (2008). Is There Intergenerational Transmission of Trauma? The Case of Combat Veterans' Children. *The American Journal of Orthopsychiatry, 78*(3), 281–289; Sangalang, C. C., & Vang, C. (2017). Intergenerational Trauma in Refugee Families: A Systematic Review. *Journal of Immigrant and Minority Health, 19*(3), 745–754; Dashorst, P., Mooren, T. M., Kleber, R. J., de Jong, P. J., & Huntjens, R. (2019). Intergenerational Consequences of the Holocaust on Offspring Mental Health: A Systematic Review of Associated Factors and Mechanisms. *European Journal of Psychotraumatology, 10*(1), 1654065.

20 Yehuda, R., & Lehrner, A. (2018). Intergenerational Transmission of Trauma Effects: Putative Role of Epigenetic Mechanisms. *World Psychiatry: Official Journal of the World Psychiatric Association (WPA), 17*(3), 243–257.

21 Lee, Y. S., Ryu, Y., Jung, W. M., Kim, J., Lee, T., & Chae, Y. (2017). Understanding Mind-Body Interaction from the Perspective of East Asian Medicine. *Evidence-Based Complementary and Alternative Medicine, Article ID 7618419*, 1–6.

22 Rushall, K. (February 21, 2019). *Chinese Medicine Treats Physical and Emotional Trauma.* Pacific College of Health and Science. Retrieved November 10, 2021, from www.pacificcollege.edu/news/blog/2014/10/05/chinese-medicine-treats-physical-and-emotional-trauma

23 Rakhee, S. (2020). Bringing People Home within Themselves. Heal from Ancestral Trauma, Depression and Burn Out. *Journal of Trauma & Acute Care, 6*(2). Insight Media Publishing. Retrieved November 10, 2021, from https://trauma-acute-care.imedpub.com/bringing-people-home-within-themselves-heal-from-ancestral-trauma-depression-burn-out.pdf

24 Woods, K., & Baruss, I. (2004). Experimental Test of Possible Psychological Benefits of Past-Life Regression. *Journal of Scientific Exploration, 18*(4), 597–608; Weiss,

B. L. (1988). *Many Lives, Many Masters: The True Story of a Prominent Psychiatrist, His Young Patient, and the Past-Life Therapy that Changed Both Their Lives.* Fireside.

25 Jain, S., Hammerschlag, R., Mills, P., Cohen, L., Krieger, R., Vieten, C., & Lutgendorf, S. (2015). Clinical Studies of Biofield Therapies: Summary, Methodological Challenges, and Recommendations. *Global Advances in Health and Medicine, 4*(Suppl), 58–66; Dale, C. (2009). *The Subtle Body: An Encyclopedia of Your Energetic Anatomy* (Illustrated ed.). Sounds True. (pp.1–21, 401–403).

26 Ornish, D., & Ornish, A. (2019). *UnDo It! How Simple Lifestyle Changes Can Reverse Most Chronic Diseases.* Ballantine Books. (p.4).

27 Colter, W. (2017). The Healing Power of Permission. *Subtle Energies Magazine*, Spring, *28*(1).

Chapter 8

1 Wahbeh, H., Yount, G., Vieten, C., Radin, D., & Delorme, A. (2020). Measuring Extraordinary Experiences and Beliefs: A Validation and Reliability Study. *F1000Research, 8*, 1741; Pretz, J. E., Brookings, J. B., Carlson, L. A., Humbert, T. K., Roy, M., Jones, M., & Memmert, D. (2014). Development and Validation of a New Measure of Intuition: The Types of Intuition Scale. *Journal of Behavioral Decision-Making, 27*(5), 454–467.

2 Lufityanto, G., Donkin, C., & Pearson, J. (2016). Measuring Intuition: Nonconscious Emotional Information Boosts Decision Accuracy and Confidence. *Psychological Science, 27*(5), 622–634.

3 Jacobsen, A. (2017). *Phenomena: The Secret History of the U.S. Government's Investigations into Extrasensory Perception and Psychokinesis* (Unabridged ed.). Little, Brown & Company. (pp.380–381).

4 Puchalski, C. M., Blatt, B., Kogan, M., & Butler, A.

(2014). Spirituality and Health. *Academic Medicine*, *89*(1), 10–16.

5   Gecewicz, C. (October, 2018). *'New Age' Beliefs Common among Both Religious and Nonreligious Americans*. Pew Research Center. www.pewresearch.org

6   Wahbeh, H., Radin, D., Mossbridge, J., Vieten, C., & Delorme, A. (2018). Exceptional Experiences Reported by Scientists and Engineers. *Explore*, *14*(5), 329–341.

7   Evans, C. (1973). Parapsychology – What the Questionnaire Revealed. *New Scientist*, *57*, 209.

8   Bem, D. J., & Honorton, C. (1994). Does Psi Exist? Replicable Evidence for an Anomalous Process of Information Transfer. *Psychological Bulletin*, *115*(1), 4–18.

9   Gauld, A. (1968). *The Founders of Psychical Research*. Routledge & Kegan Paul. (pp.137–149).

10 Simonsen, T. G. (2020). *A Short History of (Nearly) Everything Paranormal: Our Secret Powers – Telepathy, Clairvoyance & Precognition*. Watkins Publishing. (pp.211–213).

11 The Society for Psychical Research (2021). *Journal of the Society for Psychical Research*. The Society for Psychical Research. Retrieved November 10, 2021, from www.spr.ac.uk/publicationsrecordingswebevents/journal-society-psychical-research

12 Irwin, H. J., & Watt, C. A. (2007). *An Introduction to Parapsychology* (5th ed.). McFarland & Company. (pp.51–55).

13 Rhine, J. B., & Caso, A. (2011). *E.S.P. Extra Sensory Perception*. Branden Books.

14 Krippner, S., Hickman, J., Auerhahn, N., & Harris, R. (1972). Clairvoyant Perception of Target Material in Three States of Consciousness. *Perceptual and Motor Skills*, *35*(2), 439–446.

15 Wahbeh, H., Niebauer, E., Delorme, A., Carpenter, L., Radin, D., & Yount, G. (2021). A Case Study of Extended Human Capacity Perception During Energy

Medicine Treatments Using Mixed Methods Analysis. *Explore, 17*(1), 70–78.

16 Hibbard, W. S., Worring, R. W., & Brennan, R. S. (2002). *Psychic Criminology: A Guide for Using Psychics in Investigations* (2nd ed.). Charles C Thomas Publisher, Ltd.

17 Targ, R. (2012). *The Reality of ESP: A Physicist's Proof of Psychic Abilities* (Original ed.). Quest Books.

18 Jacobsen, A. (2017). *Phenomena*. Little, Brown and Company. (pp.151–152, 155–157).

19 Ibid. (pp.166, 170, 233, 322).

20 May & Marwaha, 2018, as cited in Cheung, T., Mossbridge, J., Auerbach, L., & Radin, D. (2018). *The Premonition Code: The Science of Precognition, How Sensing the Future Can Change Your Life*. Watkins Publishing. (p.88).

21 Simonsen, T. G. (2020). *A Short History of (Nearly) Everything Paranormal: Our Secret Powers – Telepathy, Clairvoyance & Precognition*. Watkins Publishing. (p.75); Targ, R. (2012). *The Reality of ESP: A Physicist's Proof of Psychic Abilities* (Original ed.). Quest Books. (pp. 15, 19, 53, 54, 57–59, 112, 147).

22 Schwartz, S. (2001). *The Alexandria Project*. Delacourte Press.

23 Kincheloe, 2003, as cited in Dossey, L. (2013). Unbroken Wholeness: The Emerging View of Human Interconnection. *Explore: The Journal of Science and Healing, 9*, 1–8.

24 Sidler, S. (2013). How Do the Fingers See? Unconscious Perception as a Basis of Intuition. *Osteopathic Medicine, 14*(1), 14–19.

25 Jain, S., Hammerschlag, R., Mills, P., Cohen, L., Krieger, R., Vieten, C., & Lutgendorf, S. (2015). Clinical Studies of Biofield Therapies: Summary, Methodological Challenges, and Recommendations. *Global Advances in Health and Medicine, 4*(Suppl), 61.

26 Boyle, D. A. (2015). Compassion Fatigue: The Cost of Caring. *Nursing, 45*(7), 48–51.

27 Gardner, W. L., Rotella, K. N., & Nikolovski, J. (2020). Implicit Maternal Intuition Confidence Is Associated with Maternal Well-Being Across Cultures. *Frontiers in Psychology, 11.*

28 Kandasamy, N., Garfinkel, S. N., Page, L., Hardy, B., Critchley, H. D., Gurnell, M., & Coates, J. M. (2016). Interoceptive Ability Predicts Survival on a London Trading Floor. *Scientific Reports, 6*(32986).

29 Radin, D. (2017). Electrocortical Correlations between Pairs of Isolated People: A Reanalysis. *F1000Research, 6,* 676.

30 Sheldrake, R., & Smart, P. (2003). Experimental Tests for Telephone Telepathy. *Journal of the Society for Psychical Research, 67,* 184–199.

31 Sheldrake, R., & Smart, P. (2005). Testing for Telepathy in Connection with E-mails. *Perceptual and Motor Skills, 101*(3), 771–786.

32 Powers, A. R., Kelley, M. S., & Corlett, P. R. (2016). Varieties of Voice-Hearing: Psychics and the Psychosis Continuum. *Schizophrenia Bulletin, 43*(1), 84–98.

33 Barrington, M. R. (2021). *Psychometry.* PSI Encyclopedia. https://psi-encyclopedia.spr.ac.uk

34 Buchanan, J. R. (1893). *Manual of Psychometry: The Dawn of a New Civilization* (4th ed.). F. H. Hodges. (pp.3, 20, 73).

35 Ibid. (p.67).

36 Denton, W. (1988). *The Soul of Things: Psychometric Experiments for Re-Living History.* Aquarian Press.

37 Simonsen, T. G. (2020). *A Short History of (Nearly) Everything Paranormal: Our Secret Powers – Telepathy, Clairvoyance & Precognition.* Watkins Publishing. (pp.46–51); McMullen, G. (1995).

38 McMullen, G. (1995). *One White Crow.* Hampton Roads Publishing Company.

39 Stevenson, I. (1960). A Review and Analysis of Paranormal Experiences Connected with the Sinking of the *Titanic. Journal of the American Society for Psychical Research, 54*, 153–171; Premonitions of the Aberfan Disaster. *Journal of the Society for Psychical Research, 44*, 169–181; Targ, R. (2012). *The Reality of ESP: A Physicist's Proof of Psychic Abilities* (Original ed.). Quest Books. (pp.126–127).

40 Irwin, H. J., & Watt, C. A. (2007). *An Introduction to Parapsychology* (5th ed.). McFarland & Company. (p.86).

41 Kruth, J. (2021). Associative Remote Viewing for Profit: Evaluating the Importance of the Judge and the Investment Instrument. *Journal of Scientific Exploration, 35*, 13–25.

42 Smith, C., Laham, D., & Moddel, G. (2014). Stock Market Prediction Using Associative Remote Viewing by Inexperienced Remote Viewers. *Journal of Scientific Exploration, 28*(7).

43 van de Castle, R. L. (1994). *Our Dreaming Mind.* Ballantine Books. (p.364).

44 Sabini, M. (1981). Dreams as an Aid in Determining Diagnosis, Prognosis, and Attitude Towards Treatment. *Psychotherapy and Psychosomatics, 36*, 24–36; Burk, L. (2015). Warning Dreams Preceding the Diagnosis of Breast Cancer: A Survey of the Most Important Characteristics. *Explore, 11*(3), 193–198.

Chapter 9

1 Menigoz, W., Latz, T. T., Ely, R. A., Kamei, C., Melvin, G., & Sinatra, D. (2020). Integrative and Lifestyle Medicine Strategies Should Include Earthing (Grounding): Review of Research Evidence and Clinical Observations. *Explore, 16*(3), 152–160.

2 Dyer, W. W. (2009). *Everyday Wisdom for Success* (Easyread Large ed.). Hay House Inc. (p.45).

3   Giacobbi, P. R., Stewart, J., Chaffee, K., Jaeschke, A. M., Stabler, M., & Kelley, G. A. (2017). A Scoping Review of Health Outcomes Examined in Randomized Controlled Trials Using Guided Imagery. *Progress in Preventive Medicine*, *2*(7), e0010.

4   Gawain, S. (1978). *Creative Visualization* (Later Printing ed.). New World Library.

5   Hamilton, D. (2018). *How Your Mind Can Heal Your Body* (Anniversary ed.). Hay House.

6   Kaiser Permanente (2019). *Audio Meditations for Health.* Kaiser Permanente. Retrieved November 4, 2021, from https://healthy.kaiserpermanente.org/southern-california/health-wellness/podcasts/conditions-diseases; Health Journeys (n.d.). *Home Page.* Health Journeys. Retrieved November 4, 2021, from www.healthjourneys.com

7   Coué, E. (1922). *Self-Mastery through Conscious Auto-Suggestion.* Starlite Distribution.

Chapter 10

1   World Health Organization. (2021) *Constitution.* World Health Organization. Retrieved September 12, 2021, from www.who.int/about/governance/constitution

2   Langevin, H. (2021). Moving the Complementary and Integrative Health Research Field Toward Whole Person Health. *The Journal of Alternative and Complementary Medicine*, *27*(8), 623–626.

3   Ibid.

4   Mills, P. J., Barsotti, T. J., Blackstone, J., Chopra, D., & Josipovic, Z. (2020). Nondual Awareness and the Whole Person. *Global Advances in Health and Medicine*, *9*. Retrieved November 4, 2021, from https://pubmed.ncbi.nlm.nih.gov/32499967/

5   McGarey, G. T., & McCombs, A. (2020). *Living Medicine.* Waterside Productions. (p.166).

6   Thornton, L. (2013). *Whole Person Caring: An Interprofessional Model for Healing and Wellness* (1st ed.). Sigma Theta Tau International. (p.xv).

7   Thornton, L. (2021). *Awards and Recognitions*. Lucia Thornton. Retrieved September 14, 2021, from www.luciathornton.com

8   Dossey, L. (1999). *Reinventing Medicine: Beyond Mind-Body to a New Era of Healing*. HarperOne. (pp.13–35).

9   Institute of Noetic Sciences (IONS). (2021). *IONS Science Publications*. IONS. Retrieved September 12, 2021, from https://noetic.org/science/publications/

10   Trzeciak, S., & Mazzarelli, A. (2019). *Compassionomics (The Revolutionary Scientific Evidence that Caring Makes a Difference)* (1st ed.). Studer Group; Jin, J., Sklar, G. E., Min Sen Oh, V., & Li, S. C. (2008). Factors Affecting Therapeutic Compliance: A Review from the Patient's Perspective. *Therapeutics and Clinical Risk Management, 4*(1), 269–286.

11   Vogel, L. (2019). Why Do Patients Often Lie to Their Doctors? *Canadian Medical Association Journal, 191*(4), E115.

12   Pink, D. H. (2006). *A Whole New Mind: Why Right-Brainers Will Rule the Future*. (Annotated ed.). Riverhead Books. (pp.1, 246).

13   Colter, W. (June 12, 2021). *Measuring the Accuracy of Medical Intuition: A Groundbreaking Study*. [Presentation]. American Holistic Nurses Association (AHNA), 41st Annual Conference.

14   Think NPC (New Philanthropy Capital). (January 13, 2021). *Systems Change: A Guide to What It Is and How To Do It*. (p.9) Think NPC. Retrieved June 22, 2021, from www.thinknpc.org/resource-hub/systems-change-a-guide-to-what-it-is-and-how-to-do-it/

INDEX

abuse 22, 77, 97, 102

Academic Consortium for Integrative Medicine & Health 8

Academies of the Sciences and of Medicine 45

Academy of Integrative Health & Medicine (AIHM) 8, 29, 144

Academy of Parapsychology and Medicine 143

acid reflux 99–101

acquired immune deficiency syndrome (AIDS) 89

acupuncture 13, 35, 83–4

acupuncturists 12, 30, 58–9, 83–4

addiction 42

adverse childhood experience (ACE) 66, 99–104, 106–8

affirmations 138, 139

AHNA see American Holistic Nurses Association

AIDS see acquired immune deficiency syndrome

AIHM see Academy of Integrative Health & Medicine

Alaura, Wil 72–5

alcohol abuse 102

Alexander, Greta 70

Alexandra Project 115

Alexandria 115

Alexandria Project 15, 123

allergens 84

Alliance Institute for Integrative Medicine 66–7

Allison, Christine 36

allopathic medicine 18, 72

see also biomedicine (Western medicine)

Alternative and Complementary Therapies 71–2

alternative medicine 25–6

American Holistic Medical Association 50, 143

American Holistic Nurses Association (AHNA) 8, 29, 144

American Medical Association 88–9

American Society of Clinical Research 70

American Society for Psychical Research (ASPR) 110

analytical thinking 53

ancestors 120

ancient Greeks 17

Andrew Weil Center for Integrative Medicine 29

Integrative Medicine Elective Rotation (IMER) program 8

anesthesia 46

angels 120

animal magnetism (mesmerism) 43–8

antibiotics 75, 83

anxiety 97, 102

Apollo-14 mission 110

archaeology, intuitive 115, 123

Archimedes 11

Aristotle 124

arthritis 80

ASPR see American Society for Psychical Research

Assessing the Accuracy of Medical Intuition (study, 2019) 29, 58–9

Assessment, Medical Intuitive 25, 26, 39–40, 82, 147–50
Association for Research and Enlightenment (A.R.E.) 49
associative remote viewing (ARV) 124
Attig, Sheryl 61
Aung, Steven 64–5
auras (auric fields) 19, 37
    and clairvoyance 113
    color 19, 66, 113
    diagnosing health issues through 66
Ayurveda 17

back pain 41–2, 66–7, 106–7
balance, whole-body 49
Behavioural Risk Factor Surveillance System (BRFSS) 102
beliefs 26
Benor, Daniel 26, 58, 65–6
Bergson, Henri 110
Bertrand, Alexandre J. F. 44
bias 33–5, 37
    confirmation (cognitive) 34
bile duct 72
BioEnergy and Health Committee 3
biofeedback 87
biofield 15, 18–19, 21, 82–3
    analysis 37, 59, 148
    and clairvoyance 113
    and clues of energetic/physical imbalance 22–3, 26
    detecting pain in the 66–7
    disturbances/blockages in the 19, 36, 105
    and the energetic damage of trauma 98
    and illness 22
    medical intuitive assessments of 26
    see also auras (auric fields); chakra system
biomedical model 47
biomedicine (Western medicine) 18, 63–5
birth process 102–3
BMJ, The (journal) 31
body 19–20
    awareness of 127

energy systems of the see biofield
    and imbalance 21–3, 26
    mechanistic view of the 145
    and Medical Intuitive Assessments 26
    needs of the 127
    scanning 59
    whole-body balance 49
    wisdom of the messages of the 137
    see also mind–body connection
body scans, intuitive 80
Braid, James 46
brain 49, 56, 80, 151
Branson, Richard 12
breath work 87
BRFSS see Behavioural Risk Factor Surveillance System
Bruyere, Rev. Rosalyn L. 66–7
Buchanan, Joseph Rodes 122–3
Burk, Larry 33, 65
Burkmar, Lucius 48

Caliendo, Jay 71–2
CAM see Complementary and Alternative Medicine
Canada 110
cancer 74, 88–9, 102, 124
caring, heart and spirit of 144–5
Carroll, Lewis 110
case studies
    back pain 41–2, 106–7
    case for 80–4
    energetic damage 99–102
    gut problems 99–102
    hand pain 147–8
    heart problems 82–3
    hernia 80–1
    hip pain 81–2
    sinus problems 83–4
    tendinitis 21–3
Cayce, Edgar 49–50, 62, 70
Centers for Disease Control and Prevention (CDC) 102
Central Intelligence Agency (CIA) 114, 115
chakra system 19, 65
    and clairvoyance 113

and gut problems 100, 101
and Medical Intuitive Assessments 37, 148
and the solar plexus chakra 100, 101
visualization 113
Chamberlain, David B. 103
change 27, 89
Chastenet, Amand-Marie-Jacques, Marquis de Puységur 44, 45
childhood abuse 22, 97, 102
childhood experience, adverse 66, 99–104, 106–8
chiropractic medicine 18
Chlamydia 83
Chopra, Deepak 85, 89, 125
Christians 109
CIA see Central Intelligence Agency
CIH see Complementary and Integrative Health
clairalience (clear smelling/clairol faction) 121–2
clairaudience (clear hearing) 20, 73, 120–2, 125
claircognizance (clear knowing) 118–20
belief in 109–10
and Medical Intuitive Assessments 73
as most commonly used meta-sense 20
and precognition 124
and psychometry 122
clairgustance (clear tasting) 122
clairosympathy 47
clairsentience (clear feeling) 20, 116–18, 122, 125, 134
clairvoyance (clear seeing) 66–7, 112–16
belief in 109–10
Caroline Myss's use of 50
Edgar Cayce's use of 49–50
and the Medical Intuitive Assessment 21–2, 36–7, 73
and mesmerism 44, 45, 46–7
Phineas Quimby's use of 48
and precognition 125

prevalence 20
and psychometry 122
Cleopatra, palace of 15, 115
clinicians
as medical intuitives 75–8
see also doctors; physicians
Coan, Mary 72–5
Cohen, Michael H. 38
coincidence 23–4
colonics 49–50
color therapy 138, 139
Colter, Wendie 2–3
compassion 116–18
compassion fatigue 117
compassionate neutrality 117
Complementary and Alternative Medicine (CAM) 27
Complementary and Integrative Health (CIH) 27, 71
complementary medicine 25–6
see also specific practices
computerized tomography (CT) scans 72
confirmation (cognitive) bias 34
confusion 80
consciousness 79
higher 89
interconnectedness 16
quantum 89
see also subconscious
convention medicine see biomedicine
coronary bypass surgery 83
Costello, Lloyd 32, 76–7
Coué, Émile 138
coughs, stubborn 83–4
Crookes, Sir William 110
CT (computerized tomography) scans 72
Curie, Marie 110
Curie, Pierre 110
Curry, Leon 70

Davis, Andrew Jackson 46–7
death 31, 88
Deleuze, Joseph P. F. 44
Denton, William 123
depression 97, 102–3, 106–7

diagnosis 26
diagnostic errors 31
dissociation 97, 104
doctor–patient relationship 20
doctors 6, 30, 149–50
    see also clinicians; physicians
domestic violence/abuse 77, 97, 102
dopamine 91
Dossey, Barbara 55
Dossey, Larry 143, 145–6
double-blind studies 61–2
Dow Jones Industrial Average 124
dreams
    journaling 120
    lucid 8
    precognitive 124, 125
drug abuse 102
Dyer, Wayne 135
dysplasia 85–6

earthing see grounding
Eccles, Sir John 16
education, higher 78–80
educators 58–9
Einstein, Albert 10, 11
electrocardiogram 18
electroencephalogram 18
electromagnetic fields 18
Elliotson, John 46
Emerson, John Norman 123
emotional stress 104
emotions
    energetic influence 26
    and health 6–7
    negative 103
    processing 135–7
    storage in the body 147–8
empathy 116–18, 134
endocrine system 19
endorphins 91
energetic blocks 5, 19, 36, 43, 98,
    105, 148
energetic damage 98–102, 108
energetic resilience 7
energetic resistance 5
energetics 5–6
    of trauma 97–108

energy healing methods 6, 9, 13, 39,
    113, 147
energy hygiene 132–7
epigenetics 102–4, 103–4
epilepsy 124
Esdaile, James 46
ESP see extrasensory perception
essential oils 49–50
ethical considerations/practice 38–9
eureka effect 11
Europe 44, 110
evidence
    for medical intuition in healthcare
    53–67
    see also research
Ewing's sarcoma 65
exercises
    Am I Intuitive? 23–4
    Can my mind affect my body?
    131–2
    Create your healing toolkit 139
    Grounding 133
    Hearing guidance 121
    How do I feel? 118
    I know what I know 119–20
    My mind's eye 115
    Releasing 136–7
    Say hello to your body 93–5
    Shielding 134–5
    words of caution regarding 130
expanded perception, tools and skills
    for 17–23
extrasensory perception (ESP) 15, 110

Faltus, Frank J. 79–80
Faraday, Michael 11
Foissac, P. 45
forgiveness 89
Foundation for Living Medicine, The
    143
France 44, 110
Franklin, Benjamin 45
free will 125
Freud, Sigmund 102, 110
future
    creating your own 125
    of healthcare 141–52

reading the 123–5

Galbraith, Jean 66
Gauss, Carl Friedrich 11
Gawain, Shakti 138
Gentile, Maria 32
Gibran, Kahlil 109
Gladstone, William Ewart 110
Global Advances in Health and
    Medicine (journal) 142
Greenhalgh, Trisha 54
grief 22, 147–8
grounding 132, 133–4, 135, 136, 137,
    139
Guarneri Integrative Health 8
guided imagery 87, 92, 113
Gulf War 1991 114–15
"gut feelings" ("hunches") 54–6, 119
    see also claircognizance (clear
    knowing)
gut health 49, 99–102

Hamilton, David R. 138
Hammid, Hella 14–15, 114, 115
hands
    ink prints 70
    painful 147–8
Hay, Louise 8, 89–90, 116
Hay House 89
Hayden, Maria B. 47
healing
    blockages to 105–6
    quantum 85, 89
    toolkits 137–9
    see also self-healing
health
    and life force energy 17–18
    new definition of 142–6
    and the psyche 16
    whole-person 7–8, 14, 26, 87, 142
Health Journeys 138
healthcare 13
    and change 27
    disease-based model of 143
    evidence for medical intuition in
        53–67
    failures 141

future 141–52
    medical model 145
    and the mind–body connection
        85–7
    nature of 10
    new era of 69, 145–6
    overburdened status 35
    as sacred practice 145
    unnecessary costs of 31
    whole-person approach to 14
Hearst, Patty 115
heart disease 61–2, 83, 102, 124
heart failure, congestive 61–2
herbal medicine 13
hernia mesh 81
higher education 78–80
Higher Sense Perception 62
Hindu philosophy 19, 104
hip pain 81–2
HIV see human immunodeficiency
    virus
holistic approaches 13–14, 27, 34
Holmes, Ernest 49
Holmes, Oliver Wendell, Sr. 141
homeopathy 49–50
hopelessness 35, 77, 88
human energy field 19
    see also biofield
human immunodeficiency virus (HIV)
    116
"hunches" ("gut feelings") 54–6, 119
    see also claircognizance (clear
    knowing)
hypnosis 46, 62, 103
hypnotherapy 43
hypnotic regression 104–5

ICIMH see International Congress on
    Integrative Medicine & Health
ICUs see Intensive Care Units
idiopathic conditions 86
IHPC see Integrative Health Policy
    Consortium
illness
    airborne 83
    and biofield disturbance 19
    getting to the cause of 39–40

imagery
  for grounding 133, 135
  guided 87, 92, 113
  language of 130–2
  for self-healing 137–8
  for shielding 134, 135
imagination 115, 131
immune system 49
  see also psychoneuroimmunology
indigenous peoples 104
inflammation 103, 138
influencers 51
injury, spinal 106–7
inner doctor (of the patient) 143
inner voices 120–1
inner wisdom/guidance
  see clairaudience (clear hearing)
insight 15, 54, 147–9
Institute of Medicine (IOM) 25–6
Institute of Noetic Sciences (IONS)
  109, 110–11, 113
Integrative Health Policy Consortium
  (IHPC) 3, 70–1
  BioEnergy and Health Committee 8
Integrative Health Symposium 2019
  72–3
Intensive Care Units (ICUs) 77–8,
  144, 151
intention 135
interconnectedness 16
International Congress on
  Integrative Medicine & Health
    (ICIMH) 29
intuition 1, 3
  Am I Intuitive? exercise 23–4
  and connection to your body 6–7
  definition 12
  development 8, 11–24, 109, 129,
    130
  experience of 15
  as innate quality 14–15
  marginalization 12–13
  and the meta-senses (clairs) 7, 112
  misconceptions concerning 12–14
  permeation of our lives 12
  as sixth sense 12
  taboos of 12

  transpersonal 16
  widespread belief in 109–10
  see also medical intuition
intuitive archaeology 123
intuitive assessment 43, 58
  see also Medical Intuitive Assessment
intuitive detectives 37
intuitive flashes 147–9
Intuitive IQ, assessment 127–9
IOM *see* Institute of Medicine
IONS see Institute of Noetic Sciences
irritable bowel syndrome 90
Ivy League 79–80

Jain, Shamini 103
James, William 49, 110
Jobst, Kim A. 65
Journal of Alternative and
  Complementary Medicine (JACM)
    29, 61, 63–5
Journal of Holistic Nursing 56
journal practice
  and clairaudience 121
  and claircognizance 120
  and clairsentience 118
  and the mind–body connection 95,
    132
  and permission for wellness 108
  and practitioners 84
  and tracking your intuitive moments
    24
  and visualization 116
Jung, Carl G. 12, 110

Kabat-Zinn, Jon 88
Kaiser Permanente 138
Kaptchuk, Ted 91
Karagulla, Shafica 62
Keegan, Lynn 55
Kelly, John 91
Kelvin, William Thomson, 1st Baron
  11
Ketchum, Wesley 70
kidney failure 124
kidney stones 41–2
Kiecolt-Glaser, Janice 103
Kincheloe, Larry 117

Kirlian photography 18–19
Kosslyn, Stephen 92
Kuruvilla, Abraham C. 71–2

Langevin, Helene 142
Lavater, Johann Kaspar 25
legal issues 38
L'Engle, Madeleine 5
Leskowitz, Eric 16
Liem, Torsten 56
life force energy 17–18, 43, 104
life stories 20–1
lifestyle change 89
lifestyle medicine 88–9
light 138, 139
Lighthouse of Pharos 115
Likert-scale surveys 59
Lincoln, Abraham 46
Living Medicine 143
Lodge, Sir Oliver 110
Louis XVI 45
Lyme disease 73–4, 75

"magnetic fluid" 43
magnetic resonance imaging (MRI)
    65, 66–7
magnets 49–50
massage therapists 148–9
massage therapy 13, 49–50
May, Edwin 114
MBSR see Mindfulness-Based Stress
    Reduction
medical errors 31, 35
medical intuition 2, 5–10, 14
    accuracy 28–9, 58–64
    in action 69–84
    advocates 62–3
    and bias 33–5
    brief history of 43–51
    definition 6, 25–42
    and ethical issues 38–9
    evidence for in healthcare 6, 28–9,
        53–67
    and the future of healthcare 7,
        141–52
    genetic components 57
    in higher education 78–80

how it can help 35–6
influencers 51
is it really intuition? 55–7
mastering 6
and the new paradigm of healthcare
    69–84
and new science 80–1
people in need of 40–2
and the physician–medical intuitive
    partnership 6, 70–5
pioneers of 6, 87–90
and the placebo effect 90–2
remote nature 37
and self-care 7, 127–39
tools and skills for 17–23
trailblazers 47–50
and the Western medicine paradigm
    63–5
what to expect 36–9
Medical Intuitive Assessments 25, 26,
    39–40, 82, 147–50
medical intuitives 29–30
    clinicians as 75–8
medical model 145
    reductionist nature 87–8
medicine
    advancement 12–13
    lifestyle 88–9
    mind–body 6–7, 87–90, 145
    naturopathic 18
    new era of 145–6
    and over treatment 31
    three eras of 145
    Western (biomedicine) 18, 63–5
meditation 13, 85–9
    guided 137, 138, 139
mediums 46
Mendoza-Cipollo, Marie 35
mental health issues 102, 121
mental healthcare providers 30
meridians 17
Mesmer, Franz Anton 43–4, 45
mesmerism (animal magnetism) 43–8
meta-senses (clairs) 7, 20, 21–2, 36–7,
    62, 109–25
    clairalience (clear smelling) 121–2
    clairaudience (clear hearing) 20, 73,

120–1, 125
claircognizance (clear knowing) 20,
    73,
    109–10, 118–20, 122, 124
clairgustance (clear tasting) 122
clairsentience (clear feeling) 20,
    116–18, 122, 125, 134
clairvoyance (clear seeing) 20–2,
    36–7, 48–50, 66–7, 73, 109–10,
    112–16, 122, 125
    combined 122–5
    developing 112
metaphysical experiences 8
Mickleborough, Tim 54
Mills, Paul J. 28, 29, 32, 61
mind cure 47–9
mind–body connection 47–9, 85–95,
    125, 130
    Can my mind affect my body?
    (exercise) 131–2
    intuitive 92–5
mind–body medicine 6–7, 145
    definition 87
    pioneers 87–90
mindfulness 87
Mindfulness-Based Stress Reduction
    (MBSR) 88
miracles, healing 86
Mitchell, Edgar 110
McGarey, Gladys T. 143–4
McMoneagle, Joe 114
McMullen, George 123
mold infestations 84
Monroe Institute, The 79
mother–child separation 101
MRI (magnetic resonance imaging)
    65, 66–7
Murphy, G. Donald 64–5
Murphy, Midge 38
Myss, Caroline 50, 63, 65, 70
mystery 2, 10, 16

Naparstek, Belleruth 138
National Center for Complementary
    and Integrative Health (NCCIH)
    142
National Institutes of Health (NIH)

18, 27, 64, 87
    Library of Medicine 54
    naturopathic medicine 18
negative thinking 91
"new age" beliefs 109
New Scientist (magazine) 110
New Thought movement 48–9
Nietzsche, Friedrich 127
NIH see National Institutes of Health
nocebo effect 91, 125
nonduality (nonlocal awareness) 16
nurses
    and self-care 131
    use of medical intuition 30, 55–6,
        58–9, 77–8
nutrition 13, 88
nutritional therapists 58–9

obstetricians 117
opioids 41–2
Oprah Winfrey Show, The (TV show)
    50, 51
Orloff, Judith 51
Ornish, Dean 97, 105
Osler, Sir William 69
osteopathy 18, 49–50
over treatment 31

pain
    abdominal 72
    back 41–2, 66–7, 106–7
    conscious emotional 88
    detection in the biofield 66–7
    discerning patterns in 66–7
    feeling other people's 44, 117
    hip 81–2
    shoulder 112–13
Paltrow, Gwyneth 51
Paracelsus 18, 85
paranormal 46–7, 110
parapsychology 57, 110
past life regression therapy 104–5
past lives 98
pattern recognition 56
Peale, Norman Vincent 49
perception
    expanded 17–23

extrasensory 15, 110
  Higher Sense Perception 62
  see also meta-senses (clairs)
Pew Research Center 109
phantom leaf effect 18–19
pharmacopeias, natural 49
phobias 105
physical exercise 88
"physician within" approach 143
physicians
  and lifestyle medicine 89
  and mind-body medicine 88–9
physician–medical intuitive
  partnerships 6, 70–5
  use of medical intuition 29–30,
    32–3, 54, 76–7, 145–6, 149–50
  see also clinicians; doctors
Pink, Daniel H. 150–1
placebo effect 90–2, 125
Plato 16
pneuma 17
Poincaré, Henri 53
police 113
positive affirmations 138, 139
positive psychology 49
positive thinking 88, 91
post-traumatic stress disorder (PTSD)
  97, 104
power differentials 38
Poyen, Charles 48
Practical Path® Medical Intuitive
  Training™ Practitioner Certification
  Program 9, 58–9
prana 17
precognition 110, 123–5
pregnancy 103
premonitions 124
preventive approaches 88–9
Price, Pat 114–15
prostatitis 71
psi 110
psyche 16
psychiatric education 78
psychic studies 78
psychologists, clinical 36
psychometry 122–3
psychoneuroimmunology 102–4

psychosis, steroid-induced 80
psychosomatic symptoms 41–2
psychotherapists 105
PTSD *see* post-traumatic stress disorder
Puchbauer, Diane 36
Puthoff, Hal 114
Puységur, Marquis de 44, 45

qi (chi) 17, 36, 104
quantum healing 85, 89
Quimby, Phineas Parkhurst 47–9, 125

radiologists 66
  holistic 65
Randall-May, Cay 82–3
Rank, Otto 102
"recognitions" 54
reincarnation 104
relationship breakdowns 22–3, 147–8
releasing 132, 135–7
remission, spontaneous 86
remote viewing 15, 113–15
research 6, 28–9, 53–67
resilience 7, 131, 132
respiratory disease 102
Rew Intuitive Judgment Scale (RIJS)
  56
Rhine, Joseph B. 15, 110
Rhine Research Center, The 110
Richet, Charles 110
right brain 56, 151
Robertson, Sandy 36
Robinson, Winter 79–80
Ruby Beach 1

sadness 147
Salk, Jonas 11
Scalmanini, Holly 35, 83–4
scanning (reading) 25, 26
  see also medical intuition
Schultz, Mona Lisa 51
Schwartz, Gary E. 61
Schwartz, Stephan A. 15, 115
science, new 80–1
Science of Consciousness annual
  conference 2006 61
scientific thought 53

séances 46
second sight 11
self, higher 16
self-care 7, 127–39, 145
self-doubt 121
self-healing 89, 127
self-help movement 89
self-hypnosis 113
senses 12
    see also meta-senses (clairs);
    perception
Seven Wonders of the Ancient World
    115
shamanism 104
Shealy, C. Norman 20, 50, 63, 70
Sheldrake, Rupert 119
shielding (energy technique) 132,
    134–7, 139
shoulder pain 112–13
Simonton, O. Carl 88–9, 125
Singh, Karandeep 33
sinus problems 83–4
sixth sense 12, 109, 112
    see also intuition
Society for Psychical Research (SPR)
    110, 111
Socrates 11
somnambulist trances 44–9
soul 16
    loss 104
    measure of the 122–3
separation from the body 16
soul's path 108
spies 114
Spinoza, Baruch 11
spirit guides 120
spirit mediums 46
spiritual ethics 38
Spiritualist movement 46–7
spirituality 16, 25, 142–5
SPR see Society for Psychical Research
Stanford Research Institute (SRI) 114
Star Gate Project 114–15
stem cells 81
steroid-induced psychosis 80
stomach ulcer 80

stress 83
    and Chinese medicine 104
    and epigenetics 103
    and immunity 103
    and pregnancy 103
stress reduction techniques 88
stroke 144
subconscious 57
substance abuse 102
subtle energy 18
    see also energetics; energy; life force
    energy
Swann, Ingo 114
symptoms, chronic, with normal lab
    results 34–5

Targ, Russell 15, 114
TCM see Traditional Chinese
    Medicine
telepathy 110, 119
tendinitis 21–3, 106
Tennyson, Alfred, Lord 110
terminal care 77–8
Tesla 11
testing, unnecessary 31, 72
Thornton, Lucia 143, 144–5
Thorson, Elizabeth 77–8
thought
    energetic influence 26
    and healing 86
    and health 6–7
    negative 91
    positive 88, 91
    power of 90
thyroid cancer 74
thyroid disorders 2
Time Magazine 89
toolkits, healing 137–9
Traditional Chinese Medicine (TCM)
    17, 104
trance
    hypnotic 62
    somnambulist 44–9
trauma 22
    acute 97
    chronic 97

complex 97
definition 97
energetics of 7, 97–108
and healing traditions 104–5
and the onset of medical intuition
    57
and permission for wellness 105–8
science of 102–4
and the soul's path 108
transgenerational 97, 98, 103–4
vicarious 97
tuberculosis 48
tumor 65, 80–1, 137
non-cancerous 85–6

ulcer, stomach 80
ultrasound 72
United States 15, 25–6, 27, 87, 110
    military 87, 114–15
United States Veterans Administration,
    Whole Health initiative 13–14

Valenzuela, Stephanie 81–2
van der Kolk, Bessel 98
Velianski, D. 44–5
veterans 13–14, 87
visualization 7, 130
    and the meta-senses 113, 115–16
    and the mind-body connection 86,
        88
    power of 92
    self-healing 131, 132, 137–8
vitalism 17–18
voices
    hearing 121
    inner 120–1

Wahbeh, Helané 33
wellbeing, full-spectrum 5
wellness, permission for 7, 105–8
Western medicine (biomedicine)
    paradigm 18, 63–5
Whole Person Caring approach 144
whole-body balance 49
whole-person health 7–8, 14, 26, 87,
    142

wholeness 143
Winfrey, Oprah 12
wisdom, of the body 137
Wisneki, Leonard A. 70–1
World Health Organization (WHO)
    142
worry 121

yoga 13, 87
Young, David 64–5

Zener, Karl 15, 110
Zener cards 14, 15, 110

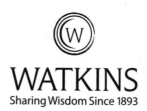

WATKINS

Sharing Wisdom Since 1893

The story of Watkins began in 1893, when scholar of esotericism John Watkins founded our bookshop, inspired by the lament of his friend and teacher Madame Blavatsky that there was nowhere in London to buy books on mysticism, occultism or metaphysics. That moment marked the birth of Watkins, soon to become the publisher of many of the leading lights of spiritual literature, including Carl Jung, Rudolf Steiner, Alice Bailey and Chögyam Trungpa.

Today, the passion at Watkins Publishing for vigorous questioning is still resolute. Our stimulating and groundbreaking list ranges from ancient traditions and complementary medicine to the latest ideas about personal development, holistic wellbeing and consciousness exploration. We remain at the cutting edge, committed to publishing books that change lives.

DISCOVER MORE AT:
www.watkinspublishing.com

Read our blog

Watch and listen to
our authors in action

Sign up to
our mailing list

We celebrate conscious, passionate, wise and happy living.
Be part of that community by visiting

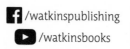 /watkinspublishing
/watkinsbooks

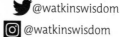 @watkinswisdom
@watkinswisdom